In Love We Trust:

The Loving Cuckold Couples Handbook

Written by Ald
Published by Dizzy-Angel Multimedia

CONTENTS

A Note to the Seekers

Welcome to those who have opened this book with curiosity, hope, or a yearning to understand themselves and others better. You are part of a remarkable community of seekers who embrace the courage to explore love, vulnerability, and authenticity in their most authentic forms.

This journey is one of self-discovery and connection. It requires a willingness to confront societal expectations, redefine intimacy for you and your partner(s), and celebrate the unique ways love can flourish when nurtured with trust and respect.

To those who find fulfillment in the delicate balance of devotion and desire, know that you are not alone and are not wrong. Your choices to honor your partner's needs and your feelings demonstrate strength, empathy, and a commitment to love that goes beyond the surface. It takes courage to embrace your authentic self and to share that truth with others.

For those who are simply curious, know that the world of loving cuckoldry is not about shame or weakness—it's about trust, communication, and the joy that comes from seeing those you love thrive. It's about celebrating the beauty of shared connection, even when that connection takes forms that might surprise or challenge conventional norms.

You are brave for seeking more—unafraid to enter a space where love, vulnerability, and trust intertwine. Whether deeply immersed in this lifestyle, just beginning to explore, or reading to understand someone you love, this book is here to guide, inspire, and honor your journey.

Take a moment to breathe deeply, open your heart, and embrace what lies ahead. This is not just a guide—it's a celebration of love in all its complexity, courage in all its forms, and the beauty of living authentically.

You are valid, worthy, and seen. In your journey, you are helping redefine love, one connection at a time.

With admiration,

Ald

Welcome to the exciting world of Cuckoldry!

Communication and Conflict Resolution in Your Dynamic

Communication is the cornerstone of trust and understanding in any relationship, and it becomes even more vital in nontraditional dynamics, such as a cuckold relationship. In a dynamic where feelings, boundaries, and desires can differ across three people, clear communication isn't just a luxury—it's an absolute necessity.

For couples in cuckold dynamics, it's not just about talking to each other; it's about genuinely listening. Everyone in the relationship must have their voice heard and their concerns validated. Hotwives, bulls, and cuckolds all have their unique feelings and experiences. The ability to express these emotions in a safe space, where each person can be vulnerable and honest, is crucial.

One essential part of communication is learning to express needs without fear of judgment. The hotwife may need to articulate what she desires physically and emotionally, while the cuckold might have insecurities or concerns that need to be voiced. Likewise, the bull may have boundaries or preferences that must be respected.

When feelings arise—whether it's happiness, anxiety, or jealousy—naming them and being able to articulate the cause is the first step to resolving any issue. Practice using "I" statements, such as "I feel hurt when..." or "I need..." rather than "You always..." or "You never..." This avoids blaming anyone and encourages a more constructive conversation.

Conflict is inevitable in any relationship but doesn't have to be destructive. In a cuckold dynamic, disputes can often arise because of insecurities, misunderstandings, or imbalances in the relationship. The key to resolution is addressing issues calmly without letting emotions spiral out of control.

When a disagreement occurs, take a step back. It's helpful to take time before responding—this can allow everyone to cool down and reflect on what's truly at the heart of the issue. Recognize that sometimes the conflict is less about the incident and more about an underlying fear or miscommunication. For instance, a cuckold might feel jealous, but that jealousy is often rooted in fear of being unworthy or not enough rather than a genuine issue with their partner's actions.

Once the immediate emotions are settled, revisit the conversation with empathy. Ask questions to understand each other's perspective truly. Instead of being defensive, approach the situation as an opportunity to understand each other better. "What do you need from me to feel secure?" or "How can we avoid this situation in the future?" These types of questions create space for healing.

Conflict resolution doesn't just happen in the heat of the moment—it's also about proactively ensuring everyone's emotional needs are met. Regular check-ins help ensure that everyone feels heard and understood. These conversations don't need to be lengthy or overly structured; they're simply about making space to discuss how the dynamic feels.

This could look like a quick discussion once a week or a more in-depth conversation after a significant experience, such as the hotwife's encounter with a bull. During these check-ins, discussing negative feelings and positives is essential—what's working well, what feels fulfilling, and what everyone is excited about. This approach prevents resentment and ensures the relationship remains fluid, adaptive, and based on mutual respect.

An essential part of communication is creating emotional safety. Every partner should feel they can express themselves without fear of rejection or judgment. This emotional safety is critical to maintaining a loving, trusting environment where people can explore their desires and vulnerabilities.

The cuckold might have moments of self-doubt or anxiety about their role, but those feelings should be met with reassurance and support. Likewise, the hotwife may have concerns about how the cuckold feels or how the bull might affect the relationship. Openly discussing these concerns and recognizing each partner's value to the dynamic is critical in fostering a secure environment.

Mutual respect is foundational. No one's feelings should be dismissed or belittled. If someone feels uncomfortable or uncertain, it's crucial to address it immediately. Validation and reassurance help keep everyone grounded in the love and respect that form the foundation of the relationship.

Active listening is one of the most powerful tools in any relationship, but it's essential in cuckold dynamics where the emotional stakes can feel higher. Active listening means hearing the spoken words and understanding the emotions behind them. It's about being fully present and giving your full attention to your partner.

To ensure understanding, practice active listening, focus on the speaker, avoid interrupting, and reflect on what you've heard. For example, a cuckold might say, "I feel like I'm not enough for you," and the hotwife might respond, "I hear you feel insecure, but I want you to know that I love you deeply and cherish the connection we have." This kind of response acknowledges the emotion and reinforces trust and security.

Non-violent communication (NVC) is an approach that can be highly beneficial for conflict resolution in cuckold dynamics. NVC focuses on expressing needs and feelings without judgment or criticism. The goal is to empower all partners to be heard and resolve conflicts to strengthen the relationship.

In an NVC framework, when an issue arises, each person identifies what they feel (emotion), expresses what need is not being met, and finally requests to address it. For instance, "I feel anxious (emotion) when I don't hear from you after a date with the bull (need). Would you be willing to text me a quick check-in when you get home? (request)." This framework avoids blame and focuses on expressing feelings and unmet needs in a non-accusatory way.

In a cuckold dynamic, communication is both a skill and an ongoing practice. The more you nurture this practice, the deeper the connection and trust will become between all parties involved. Open, honest communication is the key to resolving conflicts, reinforcing boundaries, and keeping the love flowing within your unique relationship. Always remember, the goal is not just a sexual or physical connection—but an emotional bond that is stronger than any challenge that might come your way.

Understanding and Defining Boundaries

In any relationship, boundaries are vital to creating safety and respect, and in the context of a cuckold dynamic, transparent and mutual boundaries are even more critical. Each person's boundaries reflect their emotional needs, physical comfort zones, and personal values. Confusion and hurt can arise without these boundaries being openly discussed, respected, and renegotiated when necessary. In a cuckold relationship, everyone—hotwife, bull, and cuckold—must have their boundaries clearly defined and openly communicated to ensure everyone's comfort and security.

Boundaries are the invisible lines that protect each person's emotional, mental, and physical well-being. For example, a cuckold may have boundaries related to the level of intimacy their wife shares with the bull. In contrast, the hotwife may have specific boundaries associated with the type of play or how she is treated. Each person needs to define what is acceptable and what is not.

When establishing boundaries, honesty and openness are essential. Don't assume you know someone else's boundaries; ask questions and listen carefully. The hotwife may have limits on how often she wants to be with a bull, while the cuckold may need reassurance before, during, or after those encounters to feel secure. The bull may also have personal boundaries about the type of intimacy they're comfortable with, whether physical or emotional.

The process of defining boundaries should be ongoing. As relationships evolve and experiences are shared, everyone's limits may change. Regular discussions about boundaries ensure that they remain clear and respected. It's also important to recognize that boundaries are not just about "what not to do"; they should also encompass "what is desired." For example, a cuckold may request certain behaviors or acts that make them feel secure or happy within the dynamic. These positive boundaries allow for growth and a deeper understanding of each other's needs.

Once boundaries are set, respecting them is non-negotiable. Boundaries are not flexible in intimacy, nor should they be disregarded for convenience. Respecting the boundaries of others within the cuckold dynamic is a direct expression of love and care. When boundaries are crossed, whether intentionally or accidentally, it can create discomfort, anxiety, and mistrust.

A significant part of respecting boundaries is understanding that the absence of certain boundaries doesn't imply an invitation for more. For example, just because a hotwife has expressed interest in seeing a bull regularly doesn't mean that her cuckold is obligated to do so. Each person's boundaries are unique and personal and should always be considered and cared for.

Mutual respect for boundaries can lead to greater trust and emotional intimacy, making the relationship healthier and more fulfilling for everyone involved. It allows for a deeper connection because everyone feels understood, cared for, and supported.

In a cuckold dynamic, the hotwife's physical boundaries with the bull are of utmost importance. But the cuckold also has the responsibility of ensuring the physical safety of all involved. Physical boundaries include things like safe sex practices, consent, and how far each person is willing to go in terms of intimacy. It's vital to be transparent about health concerns and implement measures to protect everyone from harm. Establishing these boundaries beforehand can help prevent miscommunications and ensure a healthy, safe experience.

Similarly, the cuckold might have physical boundaries related to his role—perhaps certain acts during play are uncomfortable for him, and these boundaries need to be communicated to the hotwife and bull. For example, he may not be comfortable participating in intimate activities during a session but might enjoy a supportive, secondary role in others.

While physical boundaries are crucial, emotional boundaries are just as important. Emotional boundaries are the limits you set to protect your heart and mind, and they are especially critical in a cuckold relationship where complex feelings are at play. Emotional boundaries relate to how much intimacy or emotional connection is shared between the hotwife, cuckold, and bull.

The cuckold, for instance, might struggle with feelings of jealousy or fear of abandonment, and these feelings may stem from perceived threats to emotional safety. In this case, the cuckold's emotional boundary could be that the hotwife or bull should avoid making any emotional connections that might threaten the cuckold's sense of security. However, these feelings should be expressed and communicated openly so that both the cuckold and hotwife understand the reasoning behind those emotional boundaries.

Emotional boundaries also include respecting the relationship's hierarchy and the unique dynamic between the couple. For instance, the cuckold must communicate his feelings with the hotwife but also respect the bond that exists between the hotwife and the bull. Similarly, the bull should recognize the cuckold's emotional role in the dynamic and avoid creating situations where either the cuckold or hotwife feels neglected or emotionally uncomfortable.

Boundaries must be negotiated as a group for the dynamic to work well. The cuckold, hotwife, and bull should engage in an ongoing dialogue about what everyone needs and expects from the relationship. This can be done through regular check-ins, discussions before and after experiences, and respectful, nonjudgmental communication.

When everyone feels heard, the boundaries can be adjusted as the relationship evolves. For example, a cuckold who is initially hesitant about certain acts might, over time, grow more comfortable with them as trust builds. Similarly, the hotwife may wish to explore new areas of intimacy as her desires evolve. In these cases, renegotiating boundaries ensures everyone stays comfortable and feels that their emotional and physical needs are being met.

The foundation of any cuckold dynamic, as with any relationship, is trust. Trust is built on the understanding that each person's boundaries will be respected and will not be coerced or manipulated into situations they disagree with. Boundaries manifest respect and trust; without them, the relationship cannot thrive.

Each partner should feel that they can express their feelings and desires without fear of overstepping or causing harm. Communicating and upholding boundaries builds trust, strengthens the connection, and provides a framework for everyone to experience pleasure and satisfaction in a safe, loving environment.

In a cuckold dynamic, establishing, communicating, and respecting boundaries is an ongoing practice that requires honesty, openness, and mutual respect. By recognizing and respecting each other's physical, emotional, and personal limits, each partner can better navigate the dynamic, build trust, and deepen their connection. Boundaries don't limit intimacy; instead, they protect and enhance it, creating a space where love and pleasure can flow freely, knowing everyone's needs are being met and respected.

The Importance of Communication and Consent

Communication is the cornerstone of connection, understanding, and respect. However, in a cuckold dynamic, where intimacy, emotions, and boundaries are often more complex, open, honest, and ongoing communication is even more essential. Consent—a mutual, enthusiastic agreement from everyone involved—is the foundation that ensures all participants feel comfortable, respected, and safe.

Clear communication is the framework for understanding each other's desires, limitations, and evolving needs. It's not just about talking; it's about listening deeply to what others say and recognizing and respecting their emotions, fears, and joys. Within a cuckold dynamic, communication should cover not only the practical aspects (such as logistics or health considerations) but also the emotional landscape of the relationship.

The hotwife, cuckold, and bull each bring their own needs and emotions to the table. For example, the cuckold may need reassurance about his role, the hotwife may want clarity about how to balance the dynamic with her partner, and the bull may seek an understanding of boundaries, both physical and emotional. Each person should feel heard and understood.

Honest communication is essential in the lead-up to any sexual encounters, where expectations and consent should be clearly stated and agreed upon. Everyone involved should feel comfortable speaking their truth and expressing discomfort or hesitation before engaging in intimate acts.

It's also crucial that communication remains a continuous dialogue. As relationships evolve, so too do needs and boundaries. What felt comfortable six months ago may need to be an essay. Likes and desires often change over time. Communicating about these channels ensures no one feels neglected, unheard, or exploited.

While communication establishes the foundation, consent keeps it solid. Consent in the cuckold dynamic is not a one-time conversation but an ongoing, fluid process. Before any encounter, all participants must explicitly agree to the activities, roles, and boundaries that will be respected during the experience.

Consent is about more than simply agreeing to participate. It includes the right to withdraw consent without feeling pressured, guilted, or coerced. Everyone must feel empowered to say "no" or "stop" at any point, whether before the experience begins or during it. Expressing discomfort or hesitation at any stage should be immediately respected. It's also vital to recognize that consent may look different for different people—just because one person is comfortable with something doesn't mean another person is ready to agree.

Additionally, consent is not limited to physical intimacy; emotional consent is just as necessary. The cuckold may feel uneasy about specific emotional dynamics between the hotwife and the bull, or the hotwife may have concerns about how the cuckold might think about her emotional connection with the bull. By having open conversations about emotional comfort levels, everyone can ensure they are emotionally on the same page, making the relationship more robust and fulfilling.

Consent also involves establishing safe words—clear terms that allow anyone to stop or adjust an encounter at any moment. A safe word serves as a way to communicate discomfort, hesitation, or a desire to change the direction of the experience and should be mutually understood and respected. This communication system creates an environment where everyone involved feels supported, protected, and valued.

Each person in the cuckold dynamic has a unique relationship with communication. The hotwife and cuckold are the primary partners, but communication with the bull is just as crucial. Open discussions between the hotwife and cuckold ensure that they stay aligned on their shared goals and emotional needs. At the same time, communication with the bull allows him to understand and respect the boundaries and desires of both the hotwife and cuckold.

For the cuckold, communication often focuses on the emotional aspects of the dynamic. He may need reassurance or guidance from his hotwife regarding her feelings toward the bull, as well as the reassurance that the love between them remains strong and intact. For the hotwife, communication is critical to managing the balance between satisfying her desires and maintaining the emotional and physical safety of both her cuckold and the bull. She may need to check in with both parties to ensure everyone is comfortable and their needs are met.

The bull, for his part, must also communicate his boundaries, desires, and comfort levels with both the hotwife and the cuckold. He is, after all, part of a mutual agreement that requires his consent and participation. Establishing trust and clarity with the bull, ensuring that his own emotional needs and boundaries are respected, is as vital as ensuring that the cuckold's and hotwife's needs are met. The bull may also provide feedback on the dynamic, discussing what works, what could be improved, and whether he feels he is fulfilling his role in the relationship.

Over time, relationships evolve, and so do needs and desires. Ongoing communication allows for the growth of the relationship. For example, a cuckold may initially struggle with feelings of jealousy or insecurity. Still, by communicating openly with his hotwife and the bull, he can learn to work through those feelings healthily. Similarly, the hotwife may discover new desires, and by discussing them with her cuckold and the bull, she can find ways to explore those desires while maintaining harmony within the relationship.

Communication allows everyone to feel heard, understood, and respected. It serves as the foundation upon which trust and intimacy are built. When communication flows freely and without fear of judgment, it creates an atmosphere where love, respect, and satisfaction can flourish. Each person's voice matters—not only in the moments of sexual exploration but also in the day-to-day interactions and decisions that shape the relationship.

Communication isn't always accessible, but a relationship like this must thrive. It can take effort to work through discomfort, challenge old patterns, and ensure everyone's needs are met. Yet, when communication is done well, it enhances everyone's experience and reinforces the deep love, respect, and trust at this dynamic's core.

In summary, communication and consent are the pillars that uphold a successful cuckold relationship. Without them, misunderstandings, resentment, and harm can creep in. When done with care, consideration, and openness, communication creates an environment where everyone feels secure, loved, and valued. It's the difference between a fulfilling, loving, and empowering dynamic and one that falls apart due to misalignment.

Consent, too, is not static—it evolves with the relationship. It's not simply about saying "yes" at the beginning of an encounter but continuously affirming and respecting each other's needs and desires. When communication and consent are at the heart of a relationship, it becomes more profound, meaningful, and connected for all involved.

Building a Healthy and Fulfilling Cuckold Dynamic

A cuckold dynamic is an intricate and nuanced relationship, one that requires understanding, patience, and a strong foundation of love and trust. At its core, this dynamic is about more than just the physical act of sharing a partner—it's about creating a healthy balance of emotional connection, respect, and mutual fulfillment for all participants involved. A successful cuckold relationship is built on understanding the roles of each partner, setting clear boundaries, and ensuring that everyone's emotional, physical, and psychological needs are met.

The cuckold's role in this dynamic is often misunderstood, but at its heart, it's about acceptance, vulnerability, and trust. The cuckold is not merely a passive observer but an active participant in creating the environment where the hotwife can thrive. He supports his partner's exploration of her desires, often finding joy in her happiness, satisfaction, and sexual fulfillment. The cuckold's pride comes not from his desires being fulfilled but from the knowledge that his partner is being loved and satisfied in ways that may not have been possible without the dynamic they share.

It's essential to recognize that a cuckold is not weak or "less than" in this dynamic. Instead, the cuckold is often a person who possesses an immense sense of emotional intelligence and self-awareness. He may be aware of his vulnerabilities, yet he understands that his place within the relationship isn't one of subjugation but of empowerment through love. The cuckold chooses to be part of this dynamic because it allows his partner to explore her full sexual and emotional potential while strengthening the bond they share.

The cuckold also plays a crucial role in maintaining the emotional health of the relationship. He helps set boundaries, ensures communication stays open and honest, and actively maintains the trust central to the dynamic's success. When feelings of jealousy, insecurity, or discomfort arise, the cuckold must be prepared to confront those emotions with openness, honesty, and the understanding that his emotional well-being is just as important as his partner's desires.

For the cuckold, consent and trust are not abstract concepts—they are essential components that keep the dynamic strong. Consent ensures that everyone's desires and boundaries are respected and that no one feels pressured or coerced into activities they are uncomfortable with. The cuckold's ability to express his needs, discuss his emotions, and offer feedback is vital to the dynamic's success.

Trust is equally essential. It allows the cuckold to feel secure in the relationship, knowing that his partner is honest, respectful, and committed to it. Without trust, the cuckold may feel anxiety or doubt, which can undermine the foundation of the entire dynamic. The cuckold needs to trust not only his partner's integrity but also the mutual respect shared between all parties involved.

While a cuckold may take pride in seeing his partner with another man, jealousy can sometimes arise, and it's natural for emotions to fluctuate in such an emotionally charged dynamic. The key to managing jealousy is communication. It's essential for the cuckold to express his feelings openly and for the hotwife and bull to be understanding and compassionate in their responses. When jealousy arises, it's an opportunity for growth—individually and as a relationship.

Jealousy can often stem from a place of insecurity or fear of loss, but addressing those feelings head-on through honest conversations allows the cuckold to work through them. It's important to note that jealousy doesn't diminish the love between the partners; working through jealousy can strengthen the emotional bond and reaffirm the cuckold's trust in his partner. Acknowledging and confronting jealousy can be empowering and can help the cuckold gain a deeper understanding of his feelings, needs, and desires.

Another challenge the cuckold may face is emotional complexity. Because of the intimacy and love shared within the dynamic, the cuckold may feel a range of emotions—pride, arousal, jealousy, confusion, or even sadness. These emotions are not signs of failure but rather the complexity of love and the depth of vulnerability inherent in the relationship. Working through these emotions can be cathartic, allowing for personal growth and a deeper connection with one's partner.

The cuckold is a supportive figure in the relationship, not only fulfilling a specific sexual role but also playing an essential emotional role. He helps create a safe and open space for his partner to express herself freely, whether by offering encouragement, providing emotional support, or simply being present. The cuckold understands that, in many ways, he is the emotional anchor for the hotwife.

By being there for his partner in both the challenging and joyous moments, the cuckold strengthens the emotional bond they share, allowing the hotwife to explore and express her desires fully. The cuckold's role is not about being passive but about actively supporting his partner's growth, both sexually and emotionally.

For the cuckold dynamic to thrive, the cuckold must also understand the importance of respecting the bull's role. While the cuckold may experience feelings of vulnerability or even discomfort during intimate moments, he must know that the bull is a mutual participant in the dynamic. The cuckold plays an essential part in ensuring that the bull's boundaries and desires are respected as well. It's not simply about what the cuckold needs but also about creating an environment where everyone involved feels comfortable and valued.

Respecting the bull's emotional needs and ensuring he feels appreciated for his role strengthens the mutual respect shared between all three participants. The cuckold should maintain open lines of communication with the bull, ensuring that everyone is on the same page regarding limits, expectations, and desires.

The cuckold dynamic is not for everyone, but for those who embrace it, it can offer a profoundly fulfilling and empowering relationship. The cuckold is an active and vital participant in the dynamic—his role is support, trust, and communication. By understanding the complexity of his emotions, honoring his boundaries, and actively participating in the shared goals of the relationship, the cuckold can create a powerful bond of mutual love and respect that enhances all aspects of his life.

Through dedication to communication, consent, and emotional support, the cuckold dynamic can be a fulfilling and transformative experience for all involved. The cuckold's role is one of profound emotional strength, vulnerability, and self-awareness, which ultimately contributes to a deeper and more meaningful connection with his partner and the bull.

Building a Lasting Connection: The Importance of Emotional Intimacy

In any relationship, emotional intimacy is often the cornerstone of its success. This is especially true for cuckold dynamics, where the bond between partners extends beyond the physical to encompass deep emotional trust, respect, and mutual understanding. The cuckold dynamic isn't merely about sexual exploration—it's a journey toward greater emotional depth, a space where each partner can experience growth, vulnerability, and profound connection.

For the cuckold, bull, and hotwife, emotional intimacy is what ultimately sustains and strengthens the dynamic. Participants' emotional well-being and connection to one another are just as important as their physical satisfaction. The dynamic can feel shallow, disconnected, and fleeting without emotional intimacy. However, when emotional closeness is nurtured and honored, it transforms the relationship into something extraordinary—an unbreakable bond of love, care, and mutual respect.

The cuckold dynamic is particularly rich in emotional intimacy because it often involves an intense level of vulnerability. The cuckold may express his emotions with more openness than he has in other relationships, revealing his fears, insecurities, and desires to his partner. Likewise, the hotwife and bull may share their vulnerabilities, whether it's the hotwife expressing her desires for exploration or the bull sharing his feelings about his role. Being vulnerable together fosters a profound connection that goes far beyond physical interactions.

Creating and maintaining emotional intimacy requires ongoing effort, honesty, and communication. Emotional closeness doesn't happen automatically—it takes work. Partners must be willing to open up, express their feelings, and listen to each other with empathy. The cuckold, bull, and hotwife must regularly check in to ensure that everyone's emotional needs are being met. Honest conversations, without judgment, are essential for maintaining that emotional closeness.

In a cuckold dynamic, this means the cuckold must feel comfortable sharing his feelings, whether he's experiencing joy, jealousy, sadness, or pride. The hotwife must feel safe in expressing her desires, both sexual and emotional. The bull also has his own unique needs, and the emotional connection with both the cuckold and the hotwife requires respect for his feelings as well. Each person must be heard and their emotions validated, strengthening their bond.

In a cuckold dynamic, emotional support isn't just about comfort; it's about growth. Each partner encourages the others to become better versions of themselves, whether emotionally, sexually, or personally. Emotional intimacy allows everyone to grow without fear of judgment, knowing they are accepted and loved.

The cuckold may find that being part of this dynamic gives him a sense of empowerment, not through submission, but through the growth of trust and emotional resilience. He learns to manage his emotions more effectively, confront feelings of jealousy, and embrace vulnerability with strength. The hotwife also experiences growth, finding confidence in her desires and feeling empowered by the love and support of her partners. The bull, too, may experience personal growth, deepening his emotional intelligence and understanding the nuances of the cuckold dynamic.

The beauty of a cuckold relationship lies in its transformative power. All parties can experience profound shifts in their relationships and personal lives by cultivating emotional intimacy. This isn't just about sexual exploration—it's about embracing the fullness of each person's emotional landscape, accepting each other's vulnerabilities, and creating a relationship dynamic based on trust, love, and mutual respect. The cuckold dynamic is unique in that it requires each partner to step out of their comfort zone and fully engage with the emotions of their loved ones. This creates a solid emotional foundation upon which lasting connections are built.

Over time, as emotional intimacy deepens, the cuckold, hotwife, and bull grow together. The initial explorations may have been about physical connection. Still, as trust and emotional closeness grow, the relationship transforms into something far more significant—a beautiful, loving, and emotionally fulfilling dynamic that offers room for everyone to thrive.

Emotional intimacy is the bedrock of any healthy relationship. In a cuckold dynamic, it becomes the anchor that holds everything together. It allows each partner to experience the relationship in its whole form and grow individually as a unit. Without emotional intimacy, the cuckold dynamic would not be possible. Still, with it, the connection between all parties flourishes in ways that transcend the physical and touch the heart of love and relationships.

Embracing the Dynamic of Love, Trust, and Respect

In a world where traditional structures often bind relationships, many seek new ways to experience love, intimacy, and connection. One such dynamic that has gained attention and sparked interest is the hotwife, cuckold, and bull relationship. But this book isn't about sensationalism or mere fantasy—it's about understanding a relationship structure rooted deeply in mutual respect, trust, and emotional intimacy.

At the heart of this dynamic is the concept of personal fulfillment. It isn't just about the physical aspect of sexuality; it's about exploring desires in a way that strengthens bonds, deepens emotional connections, and allows each participant to feel heard, respected, and loved.

The relationship between the hotwife, cuckold, and bull can look different for everyone. Still, it shares core principles that can be understood and explored in a healthy, respectful, and loving way. This book will serve as a guide to help you understand the roles, responsibilities, and emotional aspects of this dynamic, giving you the tools to embrace it, communicate effectively, and deepen your relationship.

At its core, the hotwife dynamic is built on trust, communication, and mutual respect. It is not just about sexual exploration—it is about creating an environment in which all participants feel empowered and respected in their roles.

The Hotwife is the woman who is allowed to explore her sexuality with others outside of her primary relationship. But this is not about promiscuity but connection, desire, and the freedom to explore. The hotwife's role is about authenticity—embracing her desires without judgment, knowing that her partner supports and loves her. Her role is deeply tied to communication because her satisfaction and emotional fulfillment are central to the relationship's health.

The cuckold is the husband or partner who supports the hotwife in her exploration. But the cuckold's role goes beyond simple observation—it's about trusting his partner, acknowledging his own emotions, and ensuring the relationship remains strong. The cuckold's role is to support and celebrate his partner's sexual freedom, which in turn deepens his connection to her. Selflessness and acceptance are essential in the cuckold's role, as he must constantly support his partner's growth while navigating his own emotions and desires.

The bull is the outside man who fulfills the hotwife's desires. His role is to connect with the hotwife emotionally and physically, but with the understanding that this is a mutual exchange, not about ownership or control. The bull's role requires respect for the relationship between the hotwife and her cuckold, ensuring the experience remains positive and consensual for all parties. His responsibility is to honor the boundaries set by the couple while bringing his strength and passion to the dynamic.

The hotwife, cuckold, and bull dynamic goes beyond just exploration or a "kink"—it is about creating a space for all participants to grow emotionally, spiritually, and even intellectually. It provides an opportunity for couples to:

By allowing the hotwife to explore her desires outside the marriage, all parties must rely on clear, open communication and trust. There is no room for secrecy—this dynamic requires transparency and mutual respect.

Each person in the dynamic should feel emotionally supported. The cuckold finds fulfillment in helping his partner, the bull finds joy in being a positive force in the hotwife's journey, and the hotwife feels empowered in her exploration.

This dynamic offers a new paradigm for love and sexuality, one that doesn't rely on traditional gender roles or expectations. Above all else, it is about emotional connection, fostering freedom within the relationship.

These dynamics often build stronger connections because they require honesty and vulnerability. The hotwife, cuckold, and bull must be open to new emotional experiences and adjust to evolving roles as their relationships deepen.

While these roles offer exciting opportunities for connection, they also come with essential responsibilities:

- **The Hotwife's Responsibility**: The hotwife must communicate openly with her partner and the bull. Her responsibility lies in being honest about her desires, sharing her needs, and remaining emotionally connected to her partner, mainly as she explores relationships with others. The hotwife is responsible for her emotional and physical fulfillment and must also maintain awareness of her partner's emotions and needs.

- **The Cuckold's Responsibility**: The cuckold's responsibility is to remain emotionally engaged in the relationship, even when navigating potentially challenging feelings like jealousy or insecurity. He must provide support and ensure that his partner feels loved and accepted. He is responsible for honoring the boundaries and agreements set with his partner and ensuring the dynamic remains positive for everyone involved.

- **The Bull's Responsibility**: The bull respects the couple's relationship and boundaries. He must be mindful of the cuckold's feelings and ensure that all experiences remain consensual and enjoyable for everyone. His job is to provide a safe and fulfilling experience for the hotwife while recognizing the cuckold's role and the trust he has placed in him.

How to Use This Book

This book is a guide, a resource, and a tool for anyone exploring or considering the hotwife dynamic. Whether you're just beginning your journey or have been in this relationship structure for a while, you'll find valuable insights and suggestions to help foster growth, understanding, and communication.

1. **As a Group Activity**: This book can be used by all three participants as a group activity. Read together and discuss the sections that resonate with each of you. Explore the roles and responsibilities, and use the prompts and exercises to deepen your understanding of each other's desires and needs.

2. **A Handbook for Starting Your Journey**: If you and your partner are interested in exploring this dynamic, this book serves as a handbook to help you lay the foundation. Use the exercises and practices to open up honest dialogue and to set clear boundaries before you begin.

3. **Introducing the Concept to Your Partner**: For those curious but unsure how to introduce the concept to a partner, this book provides a non-judgmental space to explore these ideas. It includes thoughtful conversation starters and exercises to help you communicate your feelings and desires in a way that prioritizes empathy and understanding.

4. **For Personal Reflection**: This book can also be used as a personal tool for reflection and growth. Whether you are a hotwife, cuckold, or bull, use the prompts to explore your feelings, desires, and boundaries as an individual, ensuring that you are always aligned with your own values and emotional needs.

Final Thoughts

This journey is one of exploration and growth. It requires honesty, vulnerability, and mutual respect. It's not always easy, but when done with love and understanding, it can profoundly transform your relationships. Whether you want to deepen your emotional intimacy, explore new facets of sexuality, or connect with your partner more authentically, this dynamic can elevate your love and connection.

Embrace it with an open heart, communicate with compassion, and always stay true to yourself and each other.

THE HOTWIFE

Welcome to the Hotwife section of this journey—an exploration of self-empowerment, connection, and the beauty of embracing your complete identity within a consensually non-monogamous dynamic. This section is dedicated to you—the hotwife—whose choices, desires, and experiences are celebrated. It is a space where you can honor yourself fully, profoundly respecting your autonomy and the trust you've built with your partner.

At the heart of the hotwife dynamic is a profound sense of mutual respect, communication, and love. It is not about seeking approval from others but finding fulfillment in your relationship and personal journey. As a hotwife, you are empowered to step into your desires and pleasures, knowing that they are valid and worth pursuing. Your happiness is not contingent on societal norms or judgments but on your sense of self-worth and respect for yourself and your partner.

The beauty of this dynamic lies in its ability to celebrate the connection between you and your partner and your individual growth, strength, and independence. Being a hotwife is about more than just exploring intimacy with others—it's about embracing and expressing your sexual and emotional desires with confidence and clarity. This section encourages you to step into your power as a woman, unafraid to explore, express, and revel in her pleasure.

Self-empowerment is critical in this journey. It means knowing your boundaries, expressing your needs with authenticity, and standing firm in your sense of self. It means permitting yourself to explore your desires without shame or guilt while respecting your partner's journey and embracing the shared experiences that this dynamic can bring. As a hotwife, you are not defined by your relationship dynamic but by the woman you are—a woman who makes conscious, empowered choices.

At the same time, **self-respect** is crucial in maintaining harmony within the relationship. By respecting yourself, you invite others to do the same. This includes honoring your body, mind, and spirit in every encounter and making decisions that align with your values and desires. You are worthy of love, respect, and care—not only from your partner but from yourself. Self-respect is not about perfection; it's about embracing who you are, the light and the shadow, and recognizing your inherent value.

In this section, you will find meditations that invite you to reflect on the deep trust you share with your partner, the joy of exploring desires, and the fulfillment that comes from living authentically. These practices are designed to help you connect more deeply with your pleasure, empower you to express your needs and boundaries, and honor the trust and love you share with your partner.

As you move through this section, reflect on the importance of maintaining power while navigating relationships. Understand that this dynamic is about *your* growth as much as shared experiences. Embrace the opportunities to strengthen your sense of self while deepening the bonds of connection with those you love and trust.

Whether you are new to the hotwife dynamic or have been walking this path for a while, remember that you are part of a larger community that celebrates and respects your choices. You are not alone in your desires, experiences, or journey toward self-empowerment. As you explore these meditations and practices, know that each step is an affirmation of your worth and your right to live a life that is fulfilling, joyful, and true to yourself.

This section celebrates the **whole of you**—your desires, self-respect, and love. It's about embracing your identity as a woman and partner and finding strength in your voice. The more you step into your power, the more space your relationship will have to thrive with love, trust, and freedom.

You deserve all the pleasure, respect, fulfillment life, and love offer. Embrace it all—your beauty, desires, and voice—and celebrate the woman you are unapologetically and entirely.

Embracing my desires and needs

Meditation:

Find a comfortable, quiet space where you can be at ease. Close your eyes and take a slow, deep breath in. Hold it for a moment, then exhale gently, releasing any tension or stress from your body. With each breath, let yourself sink deeper into a state of relaxation.

Now, begin to turn your attention inward. Bring your awareness to your heart and mind, where your desires and needs reside. It's okay to have these feelings. They are a natural part of who you are—your emotional and sexual essence.

Allow yourself to feel compassion for the desires that stir within you. You are not "wrong" for wanting what you do. You are whole, and your needs are valid. You have the right to embrace your desires with confidence and without shame. Let go of any judgment you may have placed upon yourself. Release the need for validation from anyone but yourself.

Imagine these desires as a beautiful light within you, glowing brightly. You no longer hide them. You honor them. See this light growing more robust and vibrant as you accept all you are. Your desires express your true self, and embracing them leads you to more profound joy and connection. You deserve fulfillment emotionally, physically, and sexually.

You now stand in your power, fully accepting who you are. Let this light surround you, offering you comfort and reassurance. With each breath, feel your confidence grow, knowing that your desires do not define you but empower you to live authentically and unapologetically. You can explore your needs without guilt and embrace your journey with open arms and an open heart.

Affirmation: *I embrace my desires and needs with love and acceptance. I honor my identity and permit myself to explore and express my true self without shame or fear. I am worthy of joy, love, and fulfillment.*

Practices in Action:

- **Activity 1: Self-Reflection and Acceptance:** Take a few moments to sit with your thoughts. Reflect on the desires you may have previously felt unsure or conflicted about. Write them down without judgment. As you do, permit yourself to accept these desires as part of your unique identity fully. Consider how they have shaped your life and your relationships. This is a space to affirm your right to feel the way you do.

  Tip: Focus on shifting any negative self-talk or judgment into positive affirmations. You deserve to feel secure in your desires.

- **Activity 2: Communicating Your Needs:** Discuss your desires with your partner (or a trusted friend). Share openly about what excites you and what you need emotionally or sexually. This could be part of a conversation about safely and consensually exploring these desires.

Tip: Create a space where your partner can share their needs, fostering mutual understanding and respect.

Journaling Prompt:

- *What desires or needs have I been hesitant to embrace fully? What would it look like if I allowed myself to accept and fully express them without fear of judgment? When you reflect on these desires, write about the emotions and how you can create more space for them.*

- *How do my desires enhance my sense of self and my relationships? What makes me feel empowered and confident in embracing them?*

Closing Reflection:

Take a moment to breathe deeply and feel the weight of this meditation settle in. Let the light of your desires shine brightly within you, a constant reminder that you are worthy of love, acceptance, and fulfillment in all aspects of your life. Embracing your desires opens the door to new experiences, deeper connections, and a more authentic version of yourself.

You are complete as you are. Embrace who you are and honor your unique journey. Trust that you are deserving of everything you desire and more.

Understanding the beauty of shared experiences

Meditation:

Find a quiet place where you can relax deeply. Close your eyes, and take a long, slow breath in, filling your lungs. Hold it for a moment, then gently exhale, releasing any stress or tension in your body. Allow yourself to settle into a calm state, knowing that this time is for you to reflect and connect with your inner self.

Now, focus on your relationship. Imagine the special bond you share with your partner. This relationship is built on trust, communication, and mutual respect. You are both on a journey celebrating your individuality and the shared experiences that bring you closer.

Think of a moment when you and your partner shared an intimate experience. It could be a moment of deep connection during exploration or the excitement of seeing each other happy in a new way. Whatever that moment was, hold it in your mind. See it clearly—the joy, the trust, the exhilaration. It wasn't just about the physical; the emotional connection made it special.

Understand that this experience was a gift you gave each other. The joy you feel comes from your partner's happiness and the shared emotional experience of giving and receiving pleasure. You are both co-creators in this journey, and this partnership makes the experience even more beautiful.

As you reflect on this, recognize that sharing experiences with your partner allows you to grow. It deepens your trust and intimacy, creating a bond that transcends the physical. The beauty lies in the mutual understanding, the excitement of exploration, and the sense of emotional fulfillment from sharing such intimate moments.

Feel grateful for the opportunity to share this journey with your partner. Acknowledge your trust in each other and your deep connection. This makes shared experiences beautiful: the love, respect, and joy from giving and receiving.

Affirmation: *I celebrate the beauty of shared experiences with my partner. I embrace our deep connection through trust, respect, and mutual understanding. I honor the love and joy that come from exploring and growing together.*

Practices in Action:

- **Activity 1: Reflecting on Shared Moments:** Take a few moments to reflect on a particular experience you and your partner have shared. It could be a recent memory or something from the past. What made that experience meaningful to you? How did it deepen your bond with your partner? Write about how sharing this moment brought you closer emotionally and reinforced the love and trust between you.

Tip: Focus on the emotional connection created through the experience. The physical moments are essential, but the shared emotional depth strengthens your relationship.

- **Activity 2: Building New Experiences Together:** Plan an experience to share with your partner that encourages mutual growth and exploration. It doesn't have to be a big event; it could be something as simple as a shared conversation, trying something new together, or even a quiet evening where you can be fully present with each other. The key is to nurture your connection and build a new, positive shared memory.

  Tip: Focus on making the experience meaningful and intentional. Ensure you and your partner are open and receptive to each other's needs and desires.

Journaling Prompt:

- *Think about a moment in your relationship where you felt exceptionally connected to your partner. What made that moment so special? Write about how you felt during and after the experience and what you learned about your connection with your partner.*

- *How do you feel when you share intimate experiences with your partner? What emotions arise when you see them happy or fulfilled? How does this contribute to your joy?*

Closing Reflection:

Feel the gratitude and joy from shared experiences as you sit in quiet reflection. You and your partner are co-creators of your journey, and each moment of exploration and connection is a testament to the love and trust you've built together. Remember that the beauty of shared experiences lies in the emotional depth and mutual respect that fuel your relationship.

Take a deep breath and allow the love and connection you feel to fill your entire being. You grow together With each experience, strengthening your bond and trust. You are not alone in this journey. You are partners, and your shared experiences are a beautiful reflection of the love and understanding you share.

Feeling empowered in my relationship

Meditation:

Find a comfortable space to relax, allowing yourself the time and space to focus solely on yourself. Close your eyes and take a deep breath, filling your lungs with air. Then, slowly exhale, releasing any tension or stress from your body. Let your body settle into stillness, knowing you are here to reconnect with your inner power.

Now, bring your awareness to your relationship. You are a vital, powerful part of it and deserve to feel empowered in your choices. Imagine the connection between you and your partner. It's built on mutual respect, trust, and love. Every choice you make and every boundary you set comes from confidence in your desires, needs, and worth.

Think about the times in your relationship when you have felt truly empowered. It may be a moment when you expressed your desires openly, communicated your needs, and were heard, or made a choice that honored who you are. Let these moments flood your mind, one after the other. Each of these experiences represents your strength, confidence, and ability to shape your journey.

Feel the power of knowing you have a voice in your relationship. You are not passive in your choices but an active participant, shaping the dynamic you share with your partner. Every time you express yourself authentically, you empower yourself and your relationship.

Allow this sense of empowerment to grow within you. With each breath, feel your self-worth increase, and trust that you deserve the love, respect, and fulfillment you desire. You are worthy of a relationship where you feel supported, heard, and celebrated for who you are.

Affirm to yourself that you are in control of your journey. You have the strength to choose the path that aligns with your needs and desires. Your voice, desires, and, most importantly, **you** matter in your relationship.

Affirmation: *I am empowered in my relationship. I honor my desires, needs, and boundaries and communicate them confidently. I trust in my worth and the love and respect I deserve. I actively participate in creating the dynamic that fulfills me and my partner.*

Practices in Action:

- **Activity 1: Reflecting on Your Empowerment** Spend some time reflecting on moments when you have felt empowered in your relationship. These moments might be big or small, but each one is significant. Write about these experiences and what they felt like. What did you learn about yourself in those moments? How did they strengthen your relationship?

Tip: Focus on moments where you communicated openly, expressed your desires, or made choices that reflected your strength. Celebrate these moments as powerful affirmations of your confidence.

- **Activity 2: Establishing Boundaries** One key aspect of empowerment in a relationship is knowing and expressing your boundaries. Take some time to write out your boundaries emotionally, sexually, and physically. Once you've written them, have an open conversation with your partner, ensuring your needs are heard and respected.

  Tip: Set authentic boundaries, not what you expect others to expect. Trust that these boundaries are essential for maintaining balance, respect, and empowerment in your relationship.

Journaling Prompt:

- *When have I felt truly empowered in my relationship? What made those moments so powerful? How can I create more of those experiences moving forward?*

- *What boundaries are essential to feel empowered and respected in my relationship? How do I express these boundaries to my partner in a way that fosters understanding and respect?*

Closing Reflection:

As you conclude this meditation, take a deep breath and feel the power of your self-worth. Know that you are empowered in your relationship, not because of what you do, but because of who you are. Your desires, needs, and boundaries are integral to your journey. By owning them and expressing them, you strengthen not only yourself but also your relationship.

You are an equal participant in the relationship dynamic, and your voice matters. Your empowerment is not something to be taken lightly—it is the foundation upon which a fulfilling, loving partnership can thrive. With each breath, allow that power to fill you, knowing you are worthy of everything you desire.

Celebrating my sexual freedom

Meditation:

Find a quiet and comfortable place where you can relax fully. Close your eyes and take a deep breath, filling your lungs with air. Hold it for a moment and then exhale slowly, letting go of any tension or distractions. Let your body settle into a relaxed state, knowing you can embrace who you are now.

Now, bring your focus to your sexual freedom. Imagine your desires as part of the beautiful, authentic expression of who you are. Your sexuality is a vital part of your identity, and it is something that deserves to be celebrated, not hidden. Feel the joy in knowing that you have the power to express your sexual self on your terms, free from judgment or shame.

Reflect on how you embrace and honor your desires. There is no one way to experience or express sexuality, and your freedom comes from being true to yourself. You have the right to explore your desires in a way that feels right to you and to express them with confidence and pride.

Think of moments in your life where you have celebrated your sexuality. It could be a simple acknowledgment of your desires, a time when you communicated openly with a partner or an experience where you allowed yourself to enjoy your sexual pleasure without inhibition fully. Remember these moments, and let the celebration of your sexual freedom fill you with pride and confidence.

Understand that celebrating your sexual freedom is not only about physical expression but about emotional liberation as well. It is about permitting yourself to experience pleasure, joy, and connection without guilt or shame. This is your journey, and you can choose how you walk it. Celebrate this freedom, knowing that it is a beautiful and empowering part of who you are.

Affirmation: *I celebrate my sexual freedom. I honor my desires and embrace my authentic self. I am free to express my sexuality in a way that is true to me, without shame or fear. My sexual expression is an empowering and beautiful part of my being.*

Practices in Action:

- **Activity 1: Sexual Self-Awareness:** Take some time to reflect on your desires and your journey of sexual freedom. Write about how you've come to embrace your sexuality. What parts of your sexual self do you feel most connected to? Where have you felt the most freedom to express yourself? Celebrate these aspects by acknowledging your progress in embracing your authentic desires.

  Tip: Reflect on both the emotional and physical aspects of your sexuality. Celebrate the joy, the curiosity, and the freedom you feel in these moments.

- **Activity 2: Open Communication** Sexual freedom thrives in an environment of open and honest communication. Take some time to talk to your partner about your physical and emotional desires. How can you create more space for each other to express yourselves freely? How can you celebrate and honor each other's sexual autonomy within your relationship?

  Tip: The goal is to foster a safe and non-judgmental environment where both you and your partner can be open and transparent about your sexual needs and desires.

Journaling Prompt:

- *What does sexual freedom mean to me? How do I express my desires with confidence and authenticity?*

- *When have I felt truly free to express my sexuality? How can I continue to honor and celebrate this freedom daily?*

Closing Reflection:

As you conclude this meditation, take a deep breath and let the power of your sexual freedom fill you with confidence. You have the right to express your desires in a way that is true to you. Your sexuality is a part of your authentic self, and it deserves to be celebrated without fear, guilt, or shame.

You are worthy of embracing your sexual desires, and the freedom to do so is a powerful gift. As you move forward, continue to honor your needs, celebrate your desires, and embrace the beautiful, liberating energy that comes with fully owning your sexual self.

Appreciating my husband's trust

Meditation:

Find a comfortable and quiet space where you can relax fully. Close your eyes and take a slow, deep breath, filling your lungs with fresh air. Hold the breath for a moment and then gently exhale, releasing tension. With each breath, allow your body to become more relaxed and grounded in the present moment.

Now, focus on the trust between you and your husband. Trust is the foundation of every strong relationship. It is the bond that keeps you connected, even in moments of uncertainty. As you reflect on this bond, let your heart fill with gratitude for the trust your husband has in you. This trust is not given lightly; it is a deep, unwavering belief in your connection and ability to honor each other's desires.

Think about how your husband has shown you trust, perhaps through his encouragement, openness, or support in expressing your desires and needs. His trust allows you to explore and experience your sexual freedom, knowing that he is by your side, secure in his love and confidence in you.

Recognize the strength it takes for him to entrust you with his heart, emotions, and vulnerability. This trust is a gift that should never be taken for granted. It is a mutual exchange—his trust in you mirrors the trust you place in him. This sacred balance helps create a space where both partners can grow, explore, and enjoy each other's happiness.

As you reflect on his trust, let feelings of gratitude and love fill your heart. Appreciate the strength it takes for him to be open, vulnerable, and trusting in you. You are worthy of that trust, and it strengthens the bond between you both. With each breath, feel that connection deepen.

Affirmation: *I am deeply grateful for my husband's trust in me. His trust strengthens our relationship and allows me to embrace my desires fully. I honor his vulnerability and appreciate the sacred bond we share. We create a space of love, support, and mutual respect.*

Practices in Action:

- **Activity 1: Acknowledging the Trust:** Consider how your husband has shown his trust in you. These moments may be subtle, but they are significant. Write down these moments, acknowledging the trust he has placed in you. What does his trust mean to you, and how does it impact your relationship?

  Tip: Celebrate these moments, whether through words of gratitude, a thoughtful gesture, or a simple moment of connection that acknowledges the strength of your trust.

- **Activity 2: Strengthening the Trust** Trust is a two-way street. Take a moment to reflect on how you can deepen and strengthen the trust between you and your husband. What actions or words can you offer to show your appreciation for his trust? How can you continue supporting him and building a more robust trust foundation in your relationship?

Tip: Consistent communication, honoring boundaries, and showing unwavering support for each other's needs and desires can strengthen trust.

Journaling Prompt:

- *What does my husband's trust mean to me, and how do I show appreciation for it?*

- *How can I strengthen the trust in our relationship, ensuring it remains a foundation for mutual growth and happiness?*

Closing Reflection:

As you conclude this meditation, take a deep breath, feeling the warmth of gratitude in your heart. Trust is a gift that deepens over time and is one of the most beautiful aspects of any loving relationship. Your husband's trust in you reflects the robust and loving bond you share. Honor it by nurturing it with care, open communication, and mutual respect.

Feel empowered by the knowledge that you have created a safe space where trust and love thrive. You are worthy of this trust, which strengthens your daily connection. With each breath, know you are building a resilient, deep, and everlasting love.

The joy of pleasure in all its forms

Meditation:

Find a comfortable and quiet place to settle into. Close your eyes and take a slow, deep breath, filling your lungs with air. Hold it for a moment, then gently release the breath, allowing any tension in your body to melt. With each breath, you become more relaxed, present, and connected to yourself.

Now, focus on pleasure. Pleasure is not something to be ashamed of or a fleeting moment of indulgence. It is a natural, integral part of being human and can be found in many forms—physical, emotional, mental, and spiritual. There is joy, fulfillment, and a deep sense of connection in each of these aspects.

As you sit in this quiet space, reflect on the pleasure in your life. How do you experience pleasure in its many forms? Perhaps it's the joy of shared intimacy with your husband, the pleasure of fulfilling your desires in a way that honors your boundaries, or the contentment that comes from knowing you are respecting yourself and your relationship.

Think about how the pursuit of pleasure is not an act of selfishness but an act of honoring yourself. When you voice and pursue your pleasure, you deepen your connection with your needs and the person you love. You are honoring your worth, desires, and right to feel joy in all aspects of your being.

Pleasure can also be found in emotional intimacy—shared moments of love, support, and mutual understanding. It can be found in giving and receiving, where both partners find joy not just in their satisfaction but in knowing that the other person is also fulfilled.

As you reflect, know that pleasure is not something to be hidden away or suppressed. It is a beautiful, sacred part of who you are. Allow yourself to honor and embrace it, knowing that your joy and satisfaction contribute to the health and strength of your relationship. Your pleasure is a gift to yourself and to those you love.

Affirmation: *I honor the joy of pleasure in all its forms. I respect my desires and my right to experience pleasure in ways that nurture my mind, body, and spirit. I embrace pleasure as a natural and beautiful part of my being and am worthy of experiencing it fully.*

Practices in Action:

- **Activity 1: Celebrating Sensual Pleasures:** Take a moment to reflect on the pleasures in your life that bring you joy. It might be a quiet moment of peace, the touch of your husband's hand, a favorite activity, or an intimate moment of connection. Acknowledge how these pleasures contribute to your overall well-being. Write down a few examples of how pleasure shows up daily and fulfills your mind, body, and soul.

Tip: Celebrate the little moments of joy, as they can be as powerful as more extensive experiences. Pleasure doesn't have to be big or extravagant to be meaningful.

- **Activity 2: Communicating Your Pleasures** To honor pleasure within your relationship, it's essential to communicate your desires openly and respectfully. Take time to express to your husband what gives you physical and emotional pleasure. This conversation is not about seeking perfection but fostering a deeper understanding and connection. How can you both work together to enhance the joy and pleasure you share?

  Tip: Practice sharing not only your desires but also your boundaries so that both you and your partner feel comfortable and safe exploring pleasure together.

Journaling Prompt:

- *What forms of pleasure bring me the most joy? How can I embrace and celebrate these pleasures in a way that respects myself and my relationship?*

- *How can I communicate my desires with my husband in a way that deepens our emotional and physical connection?*

Closing Reflection:

As you conclude this meditation, take a deep breath and feel the warmth of gratitude for the pleasures already a part of your life. Pleasure is not something to seek out through excess but nurture with intention, respect, and love. By honoring your desires, you contribute to the strength and joy of your relationship.

Remember, pleasure is a gift to yourself and those you love. It is not something to feel guilty about or hide from—it is something to be embraced, celebrated, and shared. As you progress, continue to recognize and honor the pleasure that flows through every aspect of your life, knowing you are worthy of experiencing joy in all its beautiful forms.

Love, intimacy, and connection

Meditation:

Begin by finding a quiet, comfortable space where you can fully relax. Gently close your eyes and take a deep, cleansing breath in. Hold it for a moment, then exhale slowly, releasing any tension. With each breath, feel your body becoming more relaxed, more at ease, and more grounded in the present moment.

Now, bring your awareness to the love between you and your husband. Love is the root of all connection, the energy that binds two people together. You share deep respect, care, and understanding, creating a foundation of trust and security.

Reflect on the moments of intimacy that have strengthened this love. Intimacy is about physical closeness and the emotional connection, shared vulnerability, and trust that allows you both to open your hearts fully. Think about the moments where you've shared your true selves, where your hearts were aligned in mutual understanding, and where you both felt indeed seen and heard.

Consider how this emotional intimacy deepens, evolving as you grow and change. It is the foundation on which all your experiences are built—the laughter, the conversations, the quiet moments, and the shared dreams. Love and intimacy create a space for both partners to flourish, be their most authentic selves, and find joy in each other's presence.

As you reflect, allow yourself to feel gratitude for your connection with your husband. This relationship is a gift that requires care, nurturing, and deep respect. It is a space to share your desires and vulnerabilities, knowing you will be met with love and understanding.

The connection between you and your husband is a living, breathing energy. It grows with each shared experience, each moment of love and intimacy. Through this connection, you find strength, security, and joy. Embrace the beauty of this bond, knowing that it is the core of everything else in your relationship.

Affirmation: *I am deeply grateful for the love, intimacy, and connection I share with my husband. Our bond is the foundation of our relationship; through it, we grow stronger and more connected daily. I honor the depth of our connection and the love between us.*

Practices in Action:

- **Activity 1: Deepening Intimacy:** Take time to reflect on a moment when you and your husband shared a profoundly intimate experience, whether physical, emotional, or spiritual. It might be a moment of deep conversation, a shared quiet evening, or a time when you truly understood each other's feelings. Write about this moment, describing the depth of your connection and how it enhanced your relationship.

Tip: Intimacy thrives in small, everyday moments of connection. Recognize the beauty of these moments, even when they seem ordinary, as they build a foundation for a lifelong bond.

- **Activity 2: Creating Shared Moments** Intimacy is nurtured by shared experiences. Consider ways to create new moments of emotional connection with your husband. Whether through a deep conversation, a shared hobby, or a quiet moment of reflection, focus on deepening the emotional bond you share. What can you do today to nurture this connection?

  Tip: Be intentional in creating space for emotional closeness, where you can be present without distractions.

Journaling Prompt:

- *What are the moments of intimacy and love I cherish most in my relationship? How do these moments deepen our connection?*

- *How can I nurture and strengthen the emotional intimacy between my husband and me to support our growth as individuals and partners?*

Closing Reflection:

As you conclude this meditation, take a moment to sit quietly with the feelings of love, intimacy, and connection that have filled your heart. Know that these qualities are the foundation of your relationship, and they create a space for both of you to grow, evolve, and find joy in each other's company.

Love and intimacy are not fleeting—they are the lasting bond that strengthens with each day. As you move forward, honor the sacred connection between you and your husband. This connection is built on trust, respect, and the willingness to be vulnerable with one another. Through it, you will continue to experience the beauty of shared love and intimacy, growing closer daily.

The beauty of mutual respect and openness

Meditation:

Begin by settling into a comfortable position. Close your eyes, and take a deep, calming breath. Inhale deeply, allowing the air to fill your lungs, and then exhale slowly, releasing any tension or distractions. Allow your body to relax and your mind to be present.

Now, bring your awareness to the concept of respect. Respect is the cornerstone of a healthy relationship. It is the acknowledgment of each other's worth, the recognition that both partners are equal in value and deserving of dignity, kindness, and care. Respect flows in both directions, allowing space for individuality while strengthening the shared bond between you and your partner.

Reflect on how you and your husband show respect to each other in your relationship. It could be through active listening, understanding, or allowing each other the space to voice desires, concerns, and feelings. Respect is not simply about outward actions but also about the internal attitude of appreciation, where you honor your partner for who they are, without judgment and with deep gratitude.

Openness is equally essential. Being open with your partner creates a space to express your true self without fear of rejection or criticism. Openness requires vulnerability and the courage to share your innermost thoughts, desires, and dreams. It is through transparency that deeper emotional intimacy is formed, creating a bond that is both safe and nurturing.

Think about how openness allows for growth as individuals and partners. When you are open, you invite your partner to know you—to see who you are, honestly. This fosters connection, trust, and a deeper understanding that strengthens the foundation of your relationship.

As you reflect, consider how you can continue cultivating mutual respect and openness in your relationship. How can you show your husband that you honor him through words, actions, thoughts, and behavior? How can you create a space where you feel safe, valued, and free to express yourselves fully?

Respect and openness create a space where love can thrive. By respecting each other's boundaries, desires, and individuality, you allow your relationship to flourish in an empowering, nurturing, and deeply fulfilling way.

Affirmation: *I honor my husband with deep respect and openness. I create a safe space where we can express our true selves, knowing that our relationship is built on mutual understanding, love, and trust. I celebrate the beauty of our connection, grounded in respect for who we are as individuals and partners.*

Practices in Action:

- **Activity 1: Practicing Active Listening:** Take time today to truly listen to your husband. Not just hear his words but truly listen to what he's expressing. Try to understand the content of his words and the emotions behind them. Show him that his voice matters to you. This simple practice of active listening fosters respect and creates a deeper emotional connection.

  Tip: Reflect on what you hear, paraphrasing his thoughts to show you understand. This can build trust and reinforce mutual respect.

- **Activity 2: Sharing a Vulnerable Moment** Share something vulnerable with your husband—an emotion, fear, or desire you haven't expressed before. Doing so with openness can deepen your intimacy and show respect for each other's vulnerabilities. Sharing creates a more profound sense of trust and understanding in your relationship.

  Tip: When sharing, create a safe and supportive space for your partner to respond. Openness is a two-way street, and mutual respect encourages both partners to be vulnerable.

Journaling Prompt:

- *What are how I show respect to my husband? How can I deepen this respect in our relationship?*

- *How can I create more openness in our relationship? How does sharing my thoughts, desires, and emotions help build a stronger bond with my husband?*

Closing Reflection:

As you conclude this meditation, take a deep breath and sit in the stillness of gratitude for the respect and openness in your relationship. Recognize that these qualities are not just a foundation for love but the building blocks that allow love to grow, evolve, and deepen.

You and your husband are equals in your relationship, each deserving of love, care, and understanding. Respect allows you both to flourish as individuals while strengthening your bond. Openness invites growth, intimacy, and a deeper connection.

Moving forward, continue to nurture these values in your relationship. By respecting each other's boundaries and desires and remaining open to one another, you create a space where love can thrive, and you are free to be your true selves.

Building emotional intimacy through trust

Meditation:

Find a quiet, comfortable place where you can fully relax. Gently close your eyes, take a deep breath in, and slowly exhale, releasing any tension from your body. Allow your body to relax with each breath you take. Let go of any distractions and center yourself in this moment of reflection.

Now, bring your awareness to the concept of trust. Trust is the foundation of emotional intimacy. It is the belief in your partner's reliability, honesty, and integrity. Trust allows both of you to be vulnerable and to share your deepest feelings and desires, knowing that your partner will honor and respect them.

Reflect on the trust that exists between you and your husband. Trust allows you to explore your desires and connect with your partner in a safe, supportive, and empowering way. Emotional intimacy is built through trust, allowing you to experience deeper connection and closeness.

Think about the moments when you have been able to share openly and honestly with your husband. These moments are precious because they are grounded in trust—the belief that you can be open with each other without fear of judgment or rejection. Consider how each moment strengthens your bond and deepens your emotional intimacy.

As you reflect, consider your role in creating and nurturing trust. Trust is a two-way street. Both partners must be committed to being trustworthy, keeping promises, and being reliable. How can you continue to nurture the trust in your relationship, ensuring that it is an ever-growing, ever-deepening aspect of your connection?

Remember, trust is not a static quality. It evolves as you grow and is reinforced through small, consistent actions. You build more trust when you are honest, open, and dependable. You create a stronger bond of trust whenever you keep your word, honor your partner's vulnerabilities, and act with integrity.

Affirmation: *I am committed to building and nurturing trust in my relationship. I honor my husband by being trustworthy, open, and honest. Our trust strengthens our emotional intimacy, and I am grateful for our deep connection.*

Practices in Action:

- **Activity 1: A Trust-Building Conversation:** Set aside time for an open and honest conversation with your husband about your feelings, desires, and concerns. Speak from the heart, knowing this conversation is grounded in mutual trust. This is an opportunity to deepen emotional intimacy by showing each other your true selves.

Tip: Be mindful of your partner's emotions and needs during the conversation. The goal is not only to express your thoughts but also to listen with empathy and understanding.

- **Activity 2: Acts of Reliability** Think of a small act you can do today that will reinforce the trust between you and your husband. It might be keeping a promise, following through on something important, or being present when you say you will be. Trust is built on these small, everyday actions that demonstrate reliability and consistency.

  Tip: Trust is built gradually through actions that demonstrate dependability. Even small moments of reliability contribute to a stronger foundation.

Journaling Prompt:

- *What moments have deepened the trust between my husband and me? How can I continue to nurture faith in our relationship?*

- *In what ways do I demonstrate trustworthiness in my relationship? What specific actions can I take to reinforce trust with my husband?*

Closing Reflection:

As you conclude this meditation, take a moment to be grateful for the trust you share with your husband. Trust is a living, breathing force in your relationship that strengthens with each act of honesty, openness, and reliability.

Trust is the gateway to emotional intimacy. Through trust, you can be vulnerable, share your true self, and experience a deep connection from being seen and understood by your partner. As you continue to nurture trust, you create a safe and supportive space where emotional intimacy can flourish.

Remember, trust is not a one-time achievement but an ongoing practice. Each action that demonstrates honesty, integrity, and reliability strengthens your bond. Continue to honor the trust in your relationship, and watch your emotional intimacy grow even more profound.

Gratitude for my husband's generosity

Meditation:

Find a quiet, comfortable space where you can fully relax. Close your eyes and take a deep, calming breath. Let the air fill your lungs, and then exhale slowly, releasing any tension or distractions. Allow your body to relax with each breath, sinking into calm and presence.

Now, bring your awareness to the concept of gratitude. Gratitude is not just an emotion but an acknowledgment of your relationship's love, kindness, and generosity. In this moment, focus on how your husband demonstrates generosity toward you.

Reflect on the many ways your husband expresses his love and generosity. This might be through his time, support, patience, or care. Consider the moments when he has gone out of his way to make you feel valued, seen, and loved. Please think of the little acts of kindness, the gestures of thoughtfulness, and his sacrifices to ensure your happiness and well-being.

How does his generosity make you feel? When he shares his love, time, and energy, it creates a sense of connection and security in your relationship. Consider how his generosity makes you feel safe, loved, and valued. Reflect on how these feelings of being cared for and appreciated contribute to your emotional and spiritual well-being.

As you continue to reflect, express your gratitude. Acknowledge how your husband's generosity has touched your life, and allow appreciation to fill your heart. Let this gratitude flow into your relationship, making it stronger and more loving.

Consider how you can express your generosity in return. When you show your husband that you value and appreciate him, it reinforces the bond of love and mutual respect between you. How can you create moments of kindness, support, and thoughtfulness that demonstrate your generosity? Reflect on how you can make him feel loved, valued, and appreciated in your relationship.

Affirmation: *I am deeply grateful for my husband's generosity. His love, time, and care make me feel valued and cherished. I honor his kindness and show my generosity in return. Our relationship is filled with love, appreciation, and mutual respect.*

Practices in Action:

- **Activity 1: A Thank-You Letter** Take a few minutes today to write a heartfelt thank-you letter to your husband. Express gratitude for his generosity and kindness and for enriching your life. This appreciation can strengthen your emotional bond and reinforce feelings of love and connection.

  Tip: Be specific. Detail the moments of generosity and care that have made you feel seen and loved.

- **Activity 2: Acts of Kindness** Do something thoughtful for your husband today—perhaps make his favorite meal, run an errand, or plan a particular activity together. Acts of kindness are a way to express your generosity and reinforce the love and connection between you.

  Tip: Small gestures of love and thoughtfulness can significantly impact a relationship. These acts of kindness show your partner that you value and appreciate them.

Journaling Prompt:

- *What are the specific ways in which my husband's generosity has touched my life? How does his kindness make me feel?*

- *How can I express my generosity and appreciation in our relationship? How can I honor his love, time, and care?*

Closing Reflection:

As you conclude this meditation, take a moment to be grateful for your husband's generosity and love. His kindness, care, and thoughtfulness create a foundation of emotional intimacy and mutual respect in your relationship.

Expressing gratitude deepens your sense of connection and reinforces the bond of love and appreciation you share. By acknowledging his generosity, you create a space of trust, respect, and support where you can continue to grow and thrive together.

Reveling in my independence and self-expression

Meditation:

Find a quiet space where you can relax and be fully present. Close your eyes and take a deep breath, allowing the air to fill your lungs. Slowly exhale, releasing any tension you may be holding onto. With each breath, feel your body relax deeper, allowing yourself to let go of any distractions and center yourself in this moment of reflection.

Now, focus on the concept of independence. Independence is not just about physical freedom—it's about owning your identity, desires, and voice. It is the ability to live authentically, express yourself fully, and pursue what brings you joy without hesitation or fear of judgment.

Reflect on how you express your independence in your relationship. Consider how you can make choices that align with your desires, values, and goals. As a hotwife, your autonomy is integral to your sense of self—whether it's the freedom to explore your sexuality, pursue your passions, or live with confidence in your choices.

Think about the moments in which you have felt free to express yourself. This could be when you've shared your desires with your husband or when you've been able to explore new experiences that bring you fulfillment. These moments of self-expression empower you, making you feel more confident, alive, and connected to your true self.

Take a moment to acknowledge the importance of your independence. It allows you to be true to yourself and your desires and makes you feel empowered and at peace in your relationship. In this independent space, you can be exactly who you are without conforming to anyone else's expectations or standards.

Self-expression is a vital part of this independence. When you express yourself authentically, you permit yourself to live fully and joyfully. Reflect on the ways you can continue to embrace self-expression in your life. Whether through your words, actions, or passions, expressing yourself freely allows your spirit to shine brightly.

Affirmation: *I embrace my independence and honor my right to live authentically. My self-expression is a beautiful reflection of who I am, and I celebrate my ability to be true to myself. I am empowered in my choices and confident in my desires.*

Practices in Action:

- **Activity 1: Embracing Your Voice** Take some time today to express yourself freely—whether through writing, art, dance, or any other form of self-expression that resonates with you. Let go of any fear or hesitation and allow yourself to create or communicate in a way that feels true to you. Celebrate your independence by embracing your voice and your creativity.

  Tip: Whether journaling, singing, drawing, or any other form of expression, this practice is about freedom. Allow yourself to feel proud of your individuality.

- **Activity 2: Setting Boundaries with Confidence** Independence is also about knowing and confidently expressing your limits. Take a moment to reflect on any boundaries you may need to reinforce in your relationships—whether they relate to sexual exploration, personal time, or emotional space. Practice setting these boundaries in a way that reflects your self-worth and autonomy.

  Tip: Boundaries are a way to honor yourself and your needs. Setting them with clarity and confidence will only strengthen your sense of independence.

Journaling Prompt:

- *In what ways do I express my independence in my relationship? How does embracing my freedom and authenticity contribute to my sense of well-being?*

- *What forms of self-expression make me feel most alive? How can I incorporate more of these into my life and my relationship?*

Closing Reflection:

As you conclude this meditation, take a moment to reflect on the beautiful power of independence and self-expression. These qualities are essential for your sense of self and for creating a fulfilling, authentic life. When you embrace your freedom, you empower yourself to live fully and confidently, free from the constraints of societal expectations.

Your self-expression reflects your true essence. By expressing yourself authentically, you connect with your innermost desires and align with your purpose. Embrace this freedom, knowing that your independence and self-expression are integral to your joy and fulfillment.

Remember, your independence is a gift—a gift you give to yourself and your relationship. When you are true to yourself, you also create space for others to be true to themselves. This mutual respect and authenticity will continue to strengthen the bond you share with your husband, allowing your relationship to flourish.

Empathy in sharing experiences

Meditation:

Find a quiet, comfortable space where you can relax and be present. Close your eyes, taking a deep breath through your nose. Hold it for a moment, then slowly exhale, releasing any tension or distractions you might be holding. With each breath, let your body relax, settling into a calm state.

Now, shift your focus to the power of empathy—the ability to truly feel and understand another person's emotions, desires, and boundaries. Empathy goes beyond simply hearing someone; it's about connecting with them on a deeper emotional level. In the context of your relationship, empathy is essential for creating a safe and trusting environment where both partners feel supported, understood, and respected.

Consider the moments when you and your husband have shared intimate or vulnerable experiences. Reflect on how empathy has played a role in those moments. Being open and mindful of each other's emotions and reactions creates an atmosphere of safety and mutual respect. These shared experiences become more meaningful because both of you are engaged in understanding one another's emotional and physical needs.

Think about the power of genuinely hearing your partner when they share their desires, feelings, or boundaries. Empathy lets you attune to their body language, words, and energy. It ensures that both of you are on the same page and that your experiences are shared in a way that respects each other's emotional states.

As you focus on empathy, ask yourself how to continue cultivating this understanding in your relationship. Are there ways in which you can be more mindful of your partner's emotional responses during intimate moments? Reflect on the importance of checking in with each other before or during an experience and afterward, ensuring that both of you feel valued and respected.

Empathy also involves checking in with yourself, being aware of your emotions and reactions, and ensuring that your desires align with your boundaries. This mindfulness will allow you to share experiences that feel safe and fulfilling, both emotionally and physically.

Affirmation: *I am deeply attuned to my husband's emotions, desires, and boundaries. I embrace empathy as the foundation of our shared experiences, ensuring we feel heard, valued, and respected. Our connection is built on mutual understanding, trust, and mindfulness.*

Practices in Action:

- **Activity 1: Mindful Communication:** Take a few moments daily to communicate with your husband. This could be a simple check-in, asking about how he's feeling emotionally or physically, or sharing your thoughts and feelings calmly and empathetically. The goal is to ensure that both of you feel heard and supported.

Tip: Use active listening techniques—maintain eye contact, nod, and offer verbal affirmations like "I understand" or "Tell me more" to show that you are fully present in the conversation.

- **Activity 2: Emotional Check-Ins During Intimacy** Before, during, or after intimate experiences, take a moment to check in with each other. Ask how your partner feels emotionally and physically, and ensure they feel comfortable expressing concerns, desires, or boundaries. This practice fosters empathy and ensures that consent and emotional well-being are maintained.

  Tip: You might ask, "How are you feeling right now?" or "Is there anything you need from me now?"

Journaling Prompt:

- *How does empathy influence my emotional and physical experiences with my husband? How can I improve my ability to understand and respond to his needs?*

- *What specific actions can I take to ensure we feel emotionally safe and valued in our relationship? How can I nurture empathy and open communication in my day-to-day interactions?*

Closing Reflection:

As you conclude this meditation, take a moment to reflect on the powerful role empathy plays in your relationship. Empathy is the bridge that connects you to your partner's emotional world, creating a space where both of you feel understood, supported, and respected. Being both attuned to each other's desires, boundaries, and emotional needs creates a more profound sense of connection and mutual fulfillment.

Empathy ensures that both partners are fully engaged in the shared experience, both emotionally and physically. By cultivating this mindfulness, you create a relationship where consent, trust, and respect are naturally present, allowing your connection to grow and thrive.

Remember that empathy is an ongoing practice requiring mindfulness, active listening, and regular check-ins. As you nurture this quality in your relationship, you will continue to deepen your emotional intimacy and create a safe, loving space for both of you to explore your desires and experiences together.

The power of vulnerability in love

Meditation:

Find a quiet and comfortable place where you can relax without distractions. Close your eyes, and take a slow, deep breath in. Hold it for a moment, then release the breath slowly, letting go of any tension or stress with the exhale. With each breath, sink deeper into the present moment, allowing yourself to feel grounded and at peace.

Now, focus on the concept of vulnerability. Vulnerability is often viewed as a source of weakness, but in the context of love and relationships, it is a source of immense strength. When you allow yourself to be vulnerable, you give your partner the gift of your true self—without masks, defenses, or pretenses. This openness creates an authentic connection where you and your partner can be fully seen and understood.

As a hotwife, embracing vulnerability can feel both empowering and intimidating. It requires the courage to express your desires and needs openly, to share your feelings and boundaries, and to trust your partner with your most intimate emotions. Vulnerability allows you to connect with your partner deeper, beyond the physical acts you may share.

Consider when you've allowed yourself to be vulnerable with your husband. Reflect on how these moments have deepened your connection and strengthened your bond. How did you feel when you shared your genuine emotions and expressed a desire or fear without judgment? These moments, though vulnerable, are often the ones that solidify trust and create a deeper emotional intimacy.

Think about how your husband responds to your vulnerability. Does he embrace your openness with empathy and understanding? When both partners can respect and honor each other's vulnerability, the relationship strengthens and creates a foundation built on mutual trust, compassion, and respect.

Reflect on when you've witnessed your husband being vulnerable with you. How did his vulnerability impact you? How did it allow you to connect more deeply with him? These moments of mutual vulnerability foster a loving relationship where both partners feel safe and valued.

As you reflect on vulnerability, remind yourself that it is not a weakness—an invitation to love more deeply, trust more fully, and connect more authentically. Embrace your vulnerability as a powerful force for love, knowing it brings you closer to your true self and partner.

Affirmation: *I embrace vulnerability as a source of strength in my relationship. By opening my heart and trusting my husband with my true self, I create more profound love and emotional intimacy. I honor my vulnerability and my husband's, knowing it strengthens our bond and deepens our connection.*

Practices in Action:

- **Activity 1: Share a Hidden Desire or Fear.** Take a moment to open up to your husband about a desire or fear you may have hidden. This could be related to your sexuality, your emotions, or any other aspect of your life. Be honest and open, and allow him to respond with empathy and understanding. Vulnerability is an invitation to trust and be trusted, so this practice encourages emotional honesty and connection.

  Tip: Choose a moment when you both have time to talk openly and ensure the space is safe and nonjudgmental. Approach the conversation with a spirit of vulnerability, knowing it will deepen your connection.

- **Activity 2: Create a Safe Space for Vulnerability** Together with your husband, create a ritual or practice that encourages open, vulnerable communication. This might include setting aside weekly time to discuss your feelings, desires, or emotional needs. Be sure to approach these conversations empathetically and constantly reassure each other that being vulnerable and open is okay.

  Tip: Reaffirm to each other that vulnerability is not a sign of weakness but deep trust and love. Let your conversations be rooted in respect, patience, and understanding.

Journaling Prompt:

- *What does vulnerability mean to me in the context of my relationship? How does embracing my vulnerability deepen my connection with my husband?*

- *How does it feel when my husband is vulnerable with me? In what ways does his openness create a stronger bond between us?*

Closing Reflection:

As you complete this meditation, take a moment to reflect on the profound power of vulnerability. Embrace the understanding that vulnerability is not a weakness but a gateway to deeper emotional connection, intimacy, and trust. When both partners are willing to open up to each other, it fosters a love built on honesty, acceptance, and mutual understanding.

Recognize that vulnerability is an ongoing practice. It requires both partners to create a safe space where each person can express their true self without fear of judgment. By honoring your vulnerability and respecting your partner, you build a foundation of trust that supports your relationship through moments of joy and challenge.

Remember that vulnerability is a strength—the key to connecting with your partner on a deeper, more authentic level. When you are open, you invite love to flow freely, creating a relationship rooted in mutual respect, trust, and emotional intimacy.

Finding fulfillment through my relationships

Meditation:

Begin by finding a quiet space to relax and be present with yourself. Close your eyes, take a deep breath, and allow your body to relax with each exhale. Let go of any tension or distractions, grounding yourself fully in the present moment.

Now, consider your relationship dynamics—your husband, your lovers, and the connections you share with them. As you reflect, notice that fulfillment does not come from just one aspect of the relationship but from the balance and emotional richness each connection brings.

Consider how your relationship with your husband fulfills you. Think about the trust, the intimacy, and how you share your lives. How do you both support each other's growth and happiness? This is the foundation of your genuine fulfillment—the emotional connection, the love you share, and the mutual respect you uphold. This bond is fulfilling because it is built on understanding, compassion, and trust.

Next, reflect on the fulfillment you experience from your lovers. They bring a different kind of pleasure and satisfaction, perhaps more physical but also emotional and psychological. How do your lovers fulfill parts of you that your husband may not, and how does this contribute to your happiness and completeness? Recognize that fulfillment is not limited to one person or one form of connection—it is about embracing and honoring the richness of multiple relationships, where all parties are respected and valued.

Now, shift your focus to yourself. How do you fulfill your own needs? How do you nurture your sense of self-worth and your emotional well-being? Recognize that fulfillment is not just about receiving from others—it's also about knowing and meeting your needs and allowing others to do the same.

As you continue to reflect, remember that fulfillment comes from the balance of love, trust, and respect that each individual contributes to the relationship. When everyone feels seen, heard, and valued, fulfillment naturally flows. Embrace the richness of these connections, knowing that they enhance your life meaningfully.

Affirmation: *I am fulfilled through the love, trust, and connection I share with my husband and lovers. I honor and respect all my relationships, knowing they contribute to my happiness and sense of completeness. I recognize that fulfillment comes from balance, mutual respect, and the care we give to each other.*

Practices in Action:

- **Activity 1: Acknowledging the Fulfillment of Each Partner:** Take some time to acknowledge the unique fulfillment each person brings to your life. Whether it's your husband, lover, or even yourself, please take a moment to appreciate how they contribute to your well-being. Write down three ways each person has fulfilled you, whether emotionally, spiritually, or physically.

Share these reflections with your husband and lover, and allow them to express their feelings of fulfillment.

Tip: Focus on the positive aspects of each connection. Recognize each relationship's value and how it enhances your overall fulfillment.

- **Activity 2: Fulfillment Through Communication** Spend time talking with your husband and lovers about what fulfillment looks like in your relationship. What are your needs and desires? How can they better support your fulfillment, and how can you do the same for them? Use this conversation to align on mutual needs and create a plan to honor these desires moving forward.

  Tip: Use this activity to deepen your emotional intimacy and strengthen your understanding of each other's needs. Ensure that the conversation is open, empathetic, and without judgment.

Journaling Prompt:

- *How do my relationships contribute to my sense of fulfillment? In what ways do my husband and lovers support my happiness and emotional well-being?*

- *How do I fulfill my needs, and how can I continue nurturing myself while nurturing my relationships?*

Closing Reflection:

As you conclude this meditation, take a moment to appreciate how your relationships bring fulfillment. Each connection—whether with your husband, your lovers, or even yourself—can potentially enrich your emotional, physical, and spiritual well-being. Remember that fulfillment is not one-sided; it results from mutual respect, understanding, and love. When all participants feel valued and supported, fulfillment grows naturally.

Reflect on how you can continue cultivating this fulfillment in your relationships, keeping the balance of care, trust, and empathy at the forefront. Fulfillment is a continuous process that requires giving and receiving with an open heart. By honoring the richness of your relationships, you create a life of deep connection, love, and happiness.

Feeling safe in my husband's love

Meditation:

Find a comfortable position to relax, allowing your body to settle into a space of ease. Take a deep breath, fill your lungs with air, and slowly exhale, letting go of any tension or distractions. With each breath, allow your body and mind to enter a calm awareness, fully present.

Now, begin to focus on the love your husband gives you. Imagine his love as a warm, comforting presence surrounding and protecting you. Reflect on the moments you've shared—when his words or actions have made you feel secure and cherished. Think about how he listens to you, respects your feelings, and supports your dreams. His love is the foundation of your emotional security.

As you reflect, let your mind bring up moments when you felt genuinely safe in his love—whether through his actions, words, or the trust you've built together. How does it feel to know he will always be there for you, no matter what? Visualize this safety as a protective shield that allows you to express yourself freely and explore your desires without fear of judgment or rejection.

Consider how this security enables you to give yourself entirely to him, knowing he is always there to support and accept you. The love he gives you creates a space where you can be vulnerable, honest, and authentic, knowing that no matter what, you are loved and valued. In this space of safety, you can share your desires, fantasies, and needs, all without fear or hesitation.

As you breathe deeply, remind yourself that your husband's love is a constant source of safety and security. Trust in this love, knowing it will always support and nurture you. Feel the sense of peace and protection from being loved deeply with each breath.

Affirmation: *I feel safe in my husband's love. His commitment and trust create a space where I can be my true self, explore my desires, and express my needs without fear. I trust his love and its security, knowing I am cherished and valued.*

Practices in Action:

- **Activity 1: Creating a Safe Space for Love** Spend some time with your husband, reflecting on how he shows you love and how you feel supported by him. Share with him what makes you feel safe in the relationship and what he does that helps you feel secure. Together, create a list of actions, words, or behaviors that reinforce this safety. Discuss how you can both continue to nurture this safe space for each other.

  Tip: Approach this conversation with openness and empathy. Expressing what makes you feel safe and secure while being attentive to his feelings and needs is essential.

- **Activity 2: Reaffirming Your Emotional Connection** Take a moment to write a letter to your husband, reaffirming the safety and security you feel in his love. Please share your thoughts on how his passion has positively impacted your emotional well-being and allowed you to explore your desires confidently. In this letter, also express gratitude for his trust, support, and the peace you feel knowing he loves you.

  Tip: This activity will deepen your emotional intimacy with your husband, fostering a sense of closeness and mutual understanding.

Journaling Prompt:

- *What does safety in love feel like for me? How does my husband make me feel secure and cherished in our relationship?*

- *How can I nurture a sense of safety in my relationship with my husband?*

Closing Reflection:

As you conclude this meditation, take a moment to appreciate your safety in your husband's love. Recognize that this sense of security is the foundation upon which you can explore, grow, and experience life together. His love creates an environment where you can be authentic, pursue your desires, and confidently express your needs.

Reflect on how this safety can be continually nurtured. Trust, open communication, and emotional intimacy are the keys to maintaining this sense of security. When both partners feel safe and supported, the relationship deepens, allowing each person to flourish and experience love fully.

Nurturing my own needs without guilt

Meditation:

Begin by finding a comfortable, quiet space where you can relax deeply. Close your eyes and take a slow, deep breath in. Imagine filling your body with calm, soothing energy as you breathe in. As you exhale, release any tension, stress, or feelings of obligation. Allow yourself to settle into this present moment, grounded and centered entirely.

Now, bring to mind the concept of nurturing your own needs. Reflect on the times when you've put your desires aside for the sake of others—whether for your husband, lovers, or family. How does it feel when you neglect your own needs for too long? Allow yourself to acknowledge those feelings, but don't judge them. Instead, focus on the idea that caring for yourself is not selfish but necessary for your well-being and those you love.

Consider how, as a hotwife, you often give a lot to your husband and lovers, sharing intimacy, trust, and connection. But, remember, your ability to offer from a place of genuine love and care requires you first to nurture yourself. Your needs are just as valid as theirs, and taking the time to fulfill your desires—whether it's time for rest, pursuing a passion, or simply doing something that brings you joy—enriches your life and relationships.

As you breathe deeply, allow yourself to feel the peace from honoring your needs. Know that it's okay to take time for yourself without feeling guilty. When you nurture your well-being, you are not taking away from others. Instead, you are replenishing yourself, allowing you to show up more fully in your relationships.

Affirmation: *I am worthy of nurturing my own needs. Taking time for myself does not diminish my love for others. I honor my desires and emotions without guilt, knowing that caring for myself makes me a more loving, present, and fulfilled partner.*

Practices in Action:

- **Activity 1: Self-Care Reflection** Spend time reflecting on your own needs. Write down three things you've been neglecting about yourself—emotional, physical, or spiritual—and how you can nurture those needs moving forward. Commit to dedicating time to these aspects of yourself, and ensure you do so without guilt.

  Tip: Self-care is necessary for maintaining healthy relationships. By tending to your needs, you can be more present and supportive of your partners.

- **Activity 2: Establish Boundaries and Self-Care Rituals** Establish a ritual or activity dedicated solely to your well-being—whether it's reading, exercising, taking a bath, or practicing mindfulness. Discuss with your husband and lovers how to create space to honor these moments without feeling guilty.

Tip: Set clear boundaries about your need for self-care, and ensure your partners respect those boundaries. This mutual understanding creates a healthier, more balanced dynamic in all your relationships.

Journaling Prompt:

- *What needs have I been neglecting, and how can I begin to fulfill them without feeling guilty?*

- *How can I make self-care a regular part of my life, and how will it benefit my relationships and emotional well-being?*

Closing Reflection:

As you conclude this meditation, reflect on how caring for your needs is an act of love for yourself and everyone in your life. You are worthy of the same care, attention, and respect that you give to others. By nurturing yourself, you deepen your sense of fulfillment and create more space to share your love and energy with your husband, lovers, and others.

Remember, self-care is not a luxury—it is necessary to maintain emotional balance and ensure you can give freely and authentically in your relationships. By honoring your needs without guilt, you strengthen your ability to love, be present, and embrace all life offers.

Building a more robust bond through shared joys

Meditation:

Begin by finding a comfortable, quiet space to sit or lie down. Close your eyes and take a deep, calming breath through your nose, filling your lungs. Slowly exhale through your mouth, releasing any tension or distractions. With each breath, allow yourself to settle more deeply into the present moment, relaxing your body and mind.

Think of the joyful moments you've shared with your husband and lovers. These moments of happiness, laughter, and connection are the threads that weave the fabric of your relationship. Reflect on the experiences that have brought you closer together—when you and your husband shared a special moment, when your lover's presence brought new excitement, or when a shared adventure brought you together.

What did those moments feel like? How did it feel to experience joy with others? Allow yourself to recall the feelings of lightness, connection, and happiness that filled those moments. These shared joys are the seeds of a deeper bond, growing stronger each time you experience them.

As you breathe, imagine these shared moments of joy creating a radiant energy that flows through you, your husband, and your lovers. Feel the warmth of this energy connecting you all, forming a stronger, more vibrant bond. Know that each joyful experience, no matter how small, strengthens the emotional ties between you and the people you care about.

Reflect on how important it is to cherish these moments of joy. They are not just fleeting pleasures—they are essential parts of the emotional foundation of your relationships. The more you share joy, the more trust and connection you build. This shared happiness nurtures an environment where love and affection can grow and flourish.

Affirmation: *I enjoy sharing moments with my husband and lovers. Our shared happiness strengthens our bond, creating deeper connection, trust, and love. I cherish these moments and recognize their power in building lasting emotional intimacy.*

Practices in Action:

- **Activity 1: Create a Shared Joy Experience** Plan a shared experience with your husband or lovers—something you can enjoy together. This could be a date night, a spontaneous adventure, or even a quiet moment of shared appreciation. The goal is to create a space where joy is at the forefront, allowing everyone involved to feel connected and engaged. Afterward, reflect on how this shared experience has brought you closer together.

  Tip: Make sure the activity is something that everyone will enjoy and feel comfortable with. It should be a moment of lightness and fun without any pressure.

- **Activity 2: Joy Journaling:** Take a moment to reflect on and journal about past moments of shared joy in your relationships. What made those experiences special? How did connecting with your husband and lovers feel in those moments? Write down how joy has strengthened your bond and how you can continue cultivating more of these moments in the future.

  Tip: As you journal, focus on the emotional and spiritual connection during those times, not just the physical or surface-level enjoyment.

Journaling Prompt:

- *What are some of the most joyful moments I've shared with my husband and lovers? How did those moments impact our connection and bond?*

- *How can I continue to create shared experiences of joy that will nurture and strengthen our emotional intimacy?*

Closing Reflection:

As you conclude this meditation, take a moment to appreciate the beauty and power of shared joy. Remember that joy is not just a fleeting emotion—it's a powerful tool that brings people closer together, fostering trust, understanding, and emotional connection. Each joyful moment you create with your husband and lovers is a building block for a more resilient and fulfilling relationship.

Reflect on how you can continue to nurture this bond through joyful experiences. As you do so, your connection will deepen, your love will expand, and your emotional intimacy will grow stronger.

Feeling supported in my choices

Meditation:

Begin by finding a comfortable position, either sitting or lying down. Close your eyes and take a deep breath through your nose, slowly filling your lungs with air. As you exhale, release any tension in your body. Continue to breathe deeply and calmly, letting your body relax more and more with each breath.

Now, reflect on your choices in your relationship dynamics—embracing the hotwife role, pursuing specific desires, or making decisions that honor your emotional needs. How does it feel to know your choices are supported by your husband, lovers, and those you care about? Feel the warmth of their understanding and acceptance. Feel the safety of knowing you are respected for being true to yourself.

In your mind's eye, imagine a situation where you make a meaningful decision—something you may have hesitated about in the past, but now, your partners fully support you. Perhaps it's exploring a new experience, setting a new boundary, or expressing a new desire. Feel the confidence that this support gives you. You are not alone in your decisions but surrounded by love and understanding.

As you breathe deeply, recognize that you are worthy of support. Your choices are valid, and your right to pursue your happiness and desires should be embraced by those who love you. Reflect on the importance of mutual respect and how this support enriches your relationship. Your bond grows more muscular when you feel supported, and your emotional connection deepens.

Affirmation: *I am worthy of support in my choices. My desires and boundaries are valid, and I am surrounded by love and acceptance. I trust in the support of my partners and honor my authenticity.*

Practices in Action:

- **Activity 1: Share Your Choices with Clarity** Have an open conversation with your husband and lovers about the choices you're making in your life. Express what is essential to you and what you need from them regarding support. This could include discussing boundaries, desires, or any decisions you're considering. Listen to their thoughts, ensuring this dialogue strengthens mutual understanding and respect.

  Tip: Approach the conversation with a spirit of openness, ensuring everyone feels heard and understood. Creating a space where each partner feels comfortable sharing their needs and receiving support is essential.

- **Activity 2: Reflect on Past Moments of Support.** Take a moment to reflect on times when you've felt genuinely supported in your relationship. What was the situation? How did their support make you feel? Write about those moments and express gratitude for the love and understanding shown.

Consider how these moments can inspire you to continue nurturing an environment of support in your relationships.

Tip: Gratitude is a powerful way to reinforce the positive dynamics in your relationship. Acknowledging and appreciating support strengthens the foundation of trust and respect.

Journaling Prompt:

- *When have I felt most supported by my husband and lovers in my personal choices? How did their support impact my sense of confidence and connection?*

- *What choices do I need to make now, and how can I communicate my needs for support in a way that fosters understanding and respect?*

Closing Reflection:

As you conclude this meditation, take a moment to appreciate the power of support in your relationships. Knowing that your partners are there for you, offering encouragement, understanding, and validation, helps you grow in confidence and authenticity. Feeling supported is essential for emotional well-being and maintaining a healthy, fulfilling relationship dynamic.

Reflect on how you can continue supporting each other in all your choices, big and small. Creating a culture of respect and love ensures that everyone feels empowered to be their authentic selves, and your emotional bonds will grow stronger.

Trusting in the balance of love and freedom

Meditation:

Find a quiet, comfortable place to sit or lie down. Close your eyes gently, and take a deep, cleansing breath in. As you breathe in, imagine breathing in calmness and clarity. As you exhale, release any tension or distractions from your mind and body. Continue to breathe deeply, allowing each breath to bring you closer to a sense of peace and groundedness.

Now, focus on your relationship with your husband and lovers. Reflect on the trust that exists between you all. Trust is the foundation upon which your emotional bond is built. As you allow yourself to feel this trust, think about how it creates a safe space for freedom to explore desires, experience joy, and express yourself fully, knowing that your partners trust you and love you.

Visualize yourself in a moment when you are freely engaging in the hotwife dynamic. Perhaps you are with a lover, or your husband supports you in an experience that brings you joy. Feel the balance of love and freedom in this moment—your husband's love and trust allowing you to explore and your lover's respect for your choices, knowing you are loved and trusted.

As you breathe deeply, recognize the strength in this balance. Love does not limit freedom; it supports it. Freedom does not diminish love; it enhances it. Both coexist harmoniously, allowing each partner to feel cherished, respected, and free to explore without fear of judgment or betrayal.

Reflect on the deep trust you have with your husband and lovers. This trust allows you to explore new experiences while feeling anchored in love. This trust is a gift, a constant reminder that you are loved and accepted exactly as you are and that the strength of your bond always supports your freedom.

Affirmation: *I trust in the balance of love and freedom. My desires are supported, and our mutual trust deepens my love for my husband and lovers. I am free to be myself and loved for who I am.*

Practices in Action:

- **Activity 1: Open Dialogue on Boundaries and Freedom** Have an open conversation with your husband and lovers about the balance of love and freedom in your dynamic. Discuss how trust allows each partner to explore desires while maintaining a sense of emotional connection. Clarify any boundaries that may exist, and ensure everyone feels supported in both their love and their freedom.

  Tip: Encourage honesty and openness. This conversation is an opportunity to reinforce trust and ensure each partner feels safe and respected.

- **Activity 2: Freedom Journal** Reflect on how you experience love and freedom in your relationship. How do you feel free to explore desires without compromising your love for your husband and lovers? Journal about moments where this balance has felt particularly strong and how you can continue to nurture it in your relationships.

  Tip: Focus on specific experiences where love and freedom coexist in harmony. By acknowledging these moments, you can create more of them in the future.

Journaling Prompt:

- *What does my relationship's balance of love and freedom look like? How does trust play a role in maintaining this balance?*

- *How can I nurture my freedom and the love I share with my husband and lovers?*

Closing Reflection:

As you finish this meditation, take a moment to appreciate the trust in your relationships. Trust is the foundation that allows love and freedom to coexist, creating a dynamic where you feel supported in your desires and actions. This balance of love and liberty enriches your relationships, deepening your emotional connection and allowing you to grow together.

Reflect on how trust continues to support the harmony between love and freedom. Trust gives you the strength to be true to yourself, knowing that you are loved, respected, and accepted exactly as you are.

Celebrating all of me in love and life

Meditation:

Find a quiet and comfortable space to settle into. Close your eyes and take a deep breath, allowing your chest and abdomen to expand with air. As you breathe in, imagine you are inhaling confidence, love, and joy. As you exhale, release any tension or judgment you may be holding onto. With each breath, allow yourself to sink deeper into relaxation and acceptance.

Now, bring your attention to your relationship with yourself—how do you feel about the woman you are? What do you think about the love you share with your husband and lovers? Reflect on the unique qualities that make you who you are: your strength, your beauty, your desires, and your capacity for love. Embrace all of it, for every part of you is worthy of celebration.

Think about the role you play in your relationship dynamic. As a hotwife, you are honored for your desires and your ability to express your sexual and emotional needs freely. Feel a deep appreciation for yourself, your body, your spirit, and your choices. You are not just a partner but a complete person deserving of love, freedom, and joy.

Celebrate your ability to love fully and give of yourself, whether with your husband, lovers, or yourself. Recognize the courage to explore your desires and the trust it takes to be vulnerable. Celebrate the unique journey that has brought you to where you are today, and know that you are supported and cherished for being unapologetically you.

Feel gratitude for your ability to create connections within yourself and others. You deserve all the love, pleasure, and joy life offers. Own your power and beauty, inside and out, and let that celebration fill you with warmth and peace.

Affirmation: *I celebrate all of myself in love and life. I embrace my desires, boundaries, strength, and beauty. I am worthy of love, joy, and freedom, and I honor the full expression of who I am.*

Practices in Action:

- **Activity 1: Self-Celebration Ritual** Create a small ritual to honor and celebrate yourself. This could include a moment of reflection where you list everything about yourself that you admire, appreciate, or love. You can write it down in a journal or say it aloud in front of a mirror. Take a moment to thank yourself for your strengths, kindness, courage, and ability to give and receive love.

  Tip: This celebration is not just about your role as a partner but about your wholeness as a person. Acknowledge everything that makes *you*, and let yourself feel proud and grateful for it.

- **Activity 2: Affirmation Practice** Incorporate affirmations into your daily routine. Repeat affirmations that reinforce your self-worth, beauty, and ability to celebrate yourself fully each day. You can write these affirmations in your journal or say them out loud as you look at yourself in the mirror. Examples might include: *"I am worthy of love and respect." "I celebrate the unique beauty within me."*

  Tip: Make these affirmations a consistent practice to nurture your self-love and confidence. Over time, you will internalize them and feel more empowered to live authentically.

Journaling Prompt:

- *What aspects of myself do I celebrate the most? How can I incorporate more celebration into my daily life and relationships?*

- *How do I feel when I embrace all parts of myself in my relationships? What does it feel like to be accepted and celebrated for the fullness of who I am?*

Closing Reflection:

As you close this meditation, remember that celebrating all of you is not just about self-love but the joy that comes from embracing your desires, boundaries, and individuality. Celebrating yourself fully invites more love, freedom, and happiness into your life and relationships.

By honoring all of who you are, you create more profound, more meaningful connections with your husband, lovers, and yourself. You are worthy of love, respect, and the space to be unapologetically you. Keep celebrating yourself—today and every day—and watch your relationships grow more robust, fulfilling, and authentic.

THE BULL

Welcome to the bull's journey, where passion, respect, and connection come together to form a dynamic that is not just about physical satisfaction but about emotional depth, trust, and mutual respect. In this section, you will explore your role in this unique relationship, recognizing the importance of empathy, understanding, and the powerful bond you share with both partners.

As the bull, you participate in a sacred dance—a role deeply rooted in trust, consent, and the joy of seeing others thrive. Your presence adds a layer of fulfillment to the dynamic, offering a space where desires are shared freely and openly and where the joy of others' pleasure becomes an integral part of your own. However, this role comes with a profound responsibility: to honor the emotional connection that sustains this relationship and to respect the trust placed in you by both the wife and the cuckold.

Throughout this section, you will reflect on your position's emotional and psychological nuances, embracing vulnerability, communication, and self-awareness. The meditations, affirmations, and practices will help you understand how to honor the connection you share with the couple and how your involvement can be a source of mutual growth, fulfillment, and joy. This is more than just an experience—it's about becoming part of a shared journey where respect, love, and openness are the cornerstones of a thriving and dynamic connection.

In this section, you'll also explore how to navigate boundaries carefully, ensuring that every interaction is built on mutual understanding. Through each meditation, you'll gain deeper insight into your role in nurturing your desires and the couple's emotional needs, creating a space where connection and respect flow freely and joyfully.

As you embrace the journey ahead, know that your role is about physical engagement and emotional connection, understanding, and deepening your bond with both partners. You will learn to celebrate the joy of shared experiences and love and to honor the unique dynamic you create together.

Honoring the connection with my partner

Meditation:

Take a deep breath and find a comfortable, relaxed position. Close your eyes, letting go of any tension in your body. With each inhale, feel the air filling your lungs; with each exhale, release any distractions or thoughts that may arise.

Now, picture yourself standing alongside your partner, the connection between you both palpable. Feel the trust and understanding that have been built over time. This connection reflects mutual respect, shared vulnerability, and open communication. You honor this bond not as something fragile but as something sacred and empowering.

Visualize your partner, not just physically but in a deep emotional space. See the love, trust, and mutual admiration that exists between you. You are not simply participants in this dynamic but co-creators of a relationship that values each other's needs, desires, and individuality.

With each breath, acknowledge how your participation strengthens this connection. Your respect for them, trust, and understanding are the pillars of this bond. Feel how your partner's trust in you empowers you to be the best version of yourself in this relationship.

Imagine communicating openly with your partner about your desires, needs, and boundaries. There is no shame in expressing what you want. Instead, there is a sense of empowerment—knowing your voice, desires, and connection are valid.

Breathe deeply, embracing the sense of unity and trust. With every exhale, let go of any doubts or insecurities. You are worthy of the love and trust in this relationship; honor it with your actions, words, and presence.

Affirmation:
"I honor the trust and love between my partner and me. Our bond is built on mutual respect, communication, and shared vulnerability. I am worthy of this connection, and I embrace it fully."

Practices in Action:

Activity 1: A Conversation of Respect

Today, sit down with your partner and discuss your relationship's emotional and physical aspects. Share openly about how you feel in this dynamic, and listen to their feelings. The goal is to create a space of mutual respect and understanding where your desires and boundaries are validated. This is an opportunity to deepen your connection further and enhance your trust.

Tip: Approach this conversation with empathy and open-mindedness. There are no right or wrong answers—this is about creating a safe space for both of you to be seen and heard.

Activity 2: Affirming Your Bond

Write a note to your partner expressing appreciation for the connection you share. Reflect on how their trust in you makes you feel valued. Acknowledge your role in emotionally supporting them, and thank them for trusting you. This can be a simple letter, a message, or even a conversation that affirms how deeply you respect and care for them.

Journaling Prompt:

Reflect on the emotional connection you share with your partner. What are the qualities of your relationship make you feel most bonded to them? How do you feel empowered by the trust and love you share? Write about a time when you felt deeply connected to your partner—what made that moment significant? How can you continue to nurture this bond and ensure that both of you feel respected and loved moving forward?

Write about your journey of open communication and mutual trust. What are the ways you can honor your partner's needs and desires while also expressing your own? What role does respect play in your relationship, and how can you continue to build it in every interaction?

Closing Reflection:

Take a deep breath and reflect on the practices and journaling prompts. Feel grounded in the understanding that your connection with your partner is built on a solid foundation of trust and respect. As you continue your journey together, remember that this bond is not just about shared moments; it's about continuously nurturing it through communication, empathy, and mutual honor. You are both essential to the relationship, and your role in supporting and loving each other strengthens your bond.

Respecting the boundaries set by the wife and cuckold

Meditation:

Take a deep breath and find a relaxed, comfortable position. Close your eyes, letting go of any tension in your body. As you breathe in deeply, feel the air filling your lungs; as you exhale, release any distractions from your mind.

Now, picture yourself in a space of deep respect and trust. You are in a relationship built on clear communication, understanding, and respect for the boundaries of all involved. See the wife and cuckold in your mind's eye, standing firm in their trust and love for one another, and know that your role is to honor and support the boundaries they've set.

Visualize the relationship dynamic, knowing these boundaries are not limitations but expressions of care and respect. The wife and cuckold's trust in you to honor their emotional and physical limits creates a safe environment where all parties can thrive. You are not here to take anything for granted; you are here to honor their desires and comfort zones with the same respect and reverence you expect for your needs.

As you breathe, consider how respecting boundaries enhances intimacy and connection in this dynamic. Boundaries reflect the love and care each person holds for the other. Acknowledging them creates a mutual respect and trust space where everyone feels heard, valued, and supported.

Now, imagine yourself communicating openly with both the wife and cuckold. Feel empowered to know you are helping create a safe, positive experience for all parties. There is no shame in discussing what feels right or wrong—this is an ongoing conversation based on empathy, trust, and the desire for everyone to feel respected and fulfilled.

Breathe deeply, honoring the sense of balance and respect that flows between you. With each exhale, feel a deeper understanding of how boundaries protect and nurture the emotional and physical connection between you all. In this space, everyone's needs are met with care and love.

Affirmation:
"I honor the boundaries set by the wife and cuckold. I respect their needs, desires, and limits, knowing that doing so strengthens our trust and connection."

Practices in Action:

Activity 1: Setting and Honoring Boundaries

Take some time today to have an open conversation with both the wife and cuckold about the boundaries in your dynamic. Discuss what feels comfortable for everyone, and listen with an open mind and heart. It's essential to communicate your needs while respecting theirs. Ensure that everyone feels heard and understood and that the boundaries are clear and agreed upon.

Tip: Approach this conversation with patience and empathy. Boundaries are not obstacles but expressions of care and respect for one another's comfort and well-being.

Activity 2: Affirming the Boundaries

Please write a letter to the wife and cuckold expressing your gratitude for their trust in you to respect their boundaries. In the letter, acknowledge the importance of clear communication and how it strengthens your bond. Let them know that you honor their needs and are committed to maintaining an environment of respect and trust.

Journaling Prompt:

Reflect on your understanding of boundaries within this dynamic. What does it feel like to honor the limits set by the wife and cuckold? How do these boundaries contribute to the relationship's overall sense of trust and connection? Write about a time when respecting someone's boundaries deepened your connection with them. What does ensuring everyone feels safe and respected in this dynamic take? How can you continue to nurture this level of respect moving forward?

Write about how you can ensure that everyone involved feels heard and understood when discussing boundaries. What steps can you take to honor your and others' needs in this relationship?

Closing Reflection:

Take a deep breath and reflect on the practices and journaling prompts. Feel grounded in the knowledge that by respecting boundaries, you are honoring the emotional and physical space each individual requires to feel safe, valued, and loved. Your role in this dynamic is maintaining balance, always ensuring mutual respect and trust are at the forefront. With each step, you strengthen the relationship and create a space where everyone can thrive and be their most authentic selves.

Celebrating mutual respect and open communication

Meditation:

Take a slow, deep breath and settle into a comfortable position. Close your eyes and feel the energy of peace filling your body with each inhale. As you exhale, release any tension or distractions, allowing yourself to be present.

Visualize yourself in a space where respect and communication flow freely. See the wife and cuckold by your side, both strong in their love and trust for one another. As you stand together, acknowledge the importance of open communication in this relationship. You are committed to understanding one another, listening deeply, and expressing your thoughts and feelings honestly and openly.

Imagine each conversation you have with the wife and cuckold as a reflection of the respect you hold for them. Your connection grows more vital when you communicate openly and share your desires, needs, and boundaries. There is no judgment here—only empathy, support, and the desire to create a space where everyone's needs are met.

As you breathe in, recognize the power of mutual respect. Every word shared and every need communicated affirms your love and trust. Respect is not just about boundaries—it is about truly seeing one another for who you are and accepting each other's unique perspectives and desires.

Now, imagine yourself engaging in a conversation with both the wife and cuckold, where everything is laid bare. There is no fear, no shame—just open, honest communication. You express your feelings, your desires, and your needs with confidence, knowing that the wife and cuckold will do the same. This conversation concerns mutual support, growth, and the goal of creating a fulfilling, loving dynamic.

Breathe deeply and feel the trust and connection growing between you. With each exhale, let go of any barriers that might prevent you from being open and honest in your communication. You are an integral part of this relationship and help strengthen the bond that ties you together through your words.

Affirmation:
"I celebrate the mutual respect and open communication we share. I honor our trust and am committed to maintaining a relationship built on honesty, empathy, and understanding."

Practices in Action:

Activity 1: Open Communication Exercise

Set aside time today for a candid, open conversation with both the wife and cuckold. This can be about anything—your desires, needs, or even just checking in on how everyone feels emotionally. Make sure that each person feels heard and understood. Encourage honesty and openness, and approach the conversation with empathy and respect for one another's perspectives.

Tip: Practice active listening. When the wife or cuckold speaks, focus entirely on what they are saying without interrupting. This demonstrates your respect and commitment to open, honest communication.

Activity 2: Writing a Respectful Message

Write a letter or message to the wife and cuckold expressing your gratitude for the open communication you share. In this message, highlight moments where their openness has made you feel valued and respected. Reflect on the strength of your bond and how communication plays a central role in nurturing that connection.

Journaling Prompt:

Reflect on how open communication and mutual respect enhance your relationship dynamic. How does it feel to communicate your desires and needs freely with the wife and cuckold? Write about a time when open communication strengthened your bond. How does mutual respect show up in your relationship? How can you continue to foster both in your interactions moving forward?

How do you feel when everyone in the relationship can be open and vulnerable? What role does communication play in ensuring everyone's emotional and physical needs are met? Explore how you can continue to create an environment of mutual respect and understanding in your relationship.

Closing Reflection:

Take a deep breath and reflect on the practices and journaling prompts. Feel a sense of gratitude for the open, respectful communication that strengthens your bond with the wife and cuckold. Through each conversation and each moment of honest exchange, you help create a relationship built on trust, empathy, and mutual understanding. Remember, your words have the power to build, strengthen, and nurture the dynamic you all share. By continuing to celebrate and practice open communication, you ensure that the foundation of your relationship remains strong, loving, and fulfilling.

Building emotional depth through shared experiences

Meditation:

Take a deep breath and find a comfortable position to relax fully. Gently close your eyes and breathe in a sense of calm with each inhale. As you exhale, release any tension or distractions, immersing yourself in the present moment.

Imagine yourself in a space filled with love, connection, and understanding. Picture the wife and cuckold beside you, each person fully engaged in the shared experience you're creating together. In this moment, you realize that your relationship is physical and deeply emotional. The emotional depth you build together is formed by the mutual experiences, trust, and respect underpinning each interaction.

Visualize yourself sharing a decisive, intimate moment with both the wife and cuckold. This moment is not defined by any one act or physical exchange but by the feelings of connection, support, and emotional fulfillment. Each time you share an experience, whether a tender conversation, a shared look, or an act of love, you add emotional depth to your bond. You are creating memories, and with each shared experience, you are growing closer, more connected, and more attuned to one another's emotional needs.

Imagine this shared experience as a single event and thread that weaves through your relationship, deepening your emotional connection over time. With every joyful or challenging experience, you are strengthening the emotional foundation you share. The wife and cuckold trust you more with each passing day, and you trust them, too. Through these shared moments, you create a space where each person can be vulnerable, honest, and fully themselves.

As you breathe in, embrace the understanding that emotional depth is not just about individual moments but the ongoing journey of connection, growth, and mutual support. Feel the warmth of love and trust between you, and know that each shared experience adds to the emotional depth of your bond.

Breathe in this sense of connection, and as you breathe out, let go of any doubts or fears that might hinder the emotional closeness you seek. You are an integral part of this relationship, and your willingness to share your heart, emotions, and experiences strengthens the dynamic.

Affirmation:
"I am committed to building emotional depth through shared experiences. With each moment we share, I grow closer to my partner and the cuckold, and together, we deepen the emotional foundation of our relationship."

Practices in Action:

Activity 1: Emotional Connection Exercise

Set aside time to engage in a shared emotional experience with both the wife and cuckold. This could be as simple as sharing a meaningful conversation or reminiscing about a moment you've shared. Focus on expressing your feelings and actively listening to the feelings of others. Allow the emotional exchange to strengthen your connection and deepen your bond.

Tip: Be present in the moment. Allow the emotions to flow freely, and embrace both the highs and the lows of the shared experience. Emotional vulnerability is critical to building depth.

Activity 2: Emotional Sharing Letter

Write a letter or message to the wife and cuckold, sharing your thoughts on how the emotional experiences you've shared have strengthened your bond. Reflect on how these moments have impacted you and allowed you to connect more deeply. Use this letter to express your gratitude for their openness and emotional availability.

Journaling Prompt:

Reflect on the emotional experiences you've shared with the wife and cuckold. How have these moments allowed you to connect on a deeper level? Write about a shared experience that brought you closer emotionally. What did it reveal about the emotional depth of your relationship, and how did it affect your connection with the wife and cuckold?

How do you feel when you are emotionally vulnerable with your wife and cuckold? What role does emotional depth play in your relationship? Explore how you can continue to foster emotional closeness and intimacy through shared experiences.

Closing Reflection:

Take a deep breath and reflect on the meditation, practices, and journaling prompts. Feel gratitude for the emotional depth cultivated through your shared experiences. Each moment of emotional connection is a building block in the foundation of trust, love, and mutual respect. Continue to embrace these experiences as they arise, knowing that with each shared moment, you are creating a relationship that is not only fulfilling physically but also emotionally enriching.

Appreciating the trust of both partners

Meditation:

Take a deep breath and find a quiet, comfortable space to relax and focus on this moment. Close your eyes gently, and bring in calm and peace with each inhale. With each exhale, release any lingering tension or distractions, allowing your mind and body to settle.

Imagine yourself surrounded by the trust and support of both the wife and the cuckold. Visualize this trust as a warm, glowing light that fills the space between you, creating a sense of safety and understanding. Feel your deep respect and appreciation for the unique trust they offer you.

As you breathe in, feel the strength of this trust. It's not just a feeling—it's a choice that both the wife and cuckold have made to believe in you and the bond you share. They trust you not only to respect their boundaries but to nurture their connection, to uphold their emotional well-being, and to create an environment where all of you can flourish.

Picture the wife's trust in you—her confidence in your role and your ability to honor the dynamic you share. You are not just a lover in this relationship; you are a part of a delicate balance, and her trust in you is a critical pillar. You can feel her support and belief in the relationship, knowing that her heart and desires are safe with you.

Now, envision the cuckold's trust in you. His willingness to share the wife he loves with you is not taken lightly. He trusts you to treat her with the respect and care she deserves, and he trusts you to honor the relationship dynamics. His trust in you allows him to let go of fears and experience joy in seeing his wife fulfilled.

Take a moment to appreciate the gravity of this trust. You are trusted for your role in the relationship and your ability to hold space for both partners. Trust is the foundation of everything, and in this moment, you honor it.

With each breath, recognize the gift of trust. It is not given lightly and requires a deep sense of responsibility. You appreciate the confidence they have placed in you to care for their hearts and desires and help build a relationship where all of you feel safe, respected, and loved.

As you breathe out, release any doubts or fears that may have arisen in the past. Let go of any worries about living up to this trust. Know that you honor their trust in you by simply being present, respectful, and faithful to your role.

Affirmation:
"I appreciate and honor the trust placed in me by both my partner and the cuckold. With each breath, I strengthen my commitment to uphold this trust and nurture our bond."

Practices in Action:

Activity 1: Trust-Building Conversation

Sit down with both the wife and cuckold and discuss what trust means to each of you. Please share your thoughts on how trust is demonstrated in the relationship and how it makes you feel. This conversation is about deepening your understanding of each other's needs, boundaries, and the emotional importance of trust. Be honest and open with your feelings, and listen to theirs with empathy and respect.

Tip: Remember, trust is built over time and through ongoing communication. Take time to express gratitude for their faith and share how it empowers you in your role.

Activity 2: Trust Affirmation Exercise

Take a moment to write down three specific ways in which you appreciate the trust given to you by both the wife and cuckold. These could be moments when you felt particularly respected or when you were able to help nurture their relationship. Use this to remind yourself of the profound responsibility and privilege that trust brings and how you can continue to honor it.

Journaling Prompt:

Reflect on the trust that has been extended to you in this dynamic. How do you feel when you think about the wife and cuckold trusting you with their hearts and desires? In what ways has this trust enriched your relationship? Write about a moment when you truly felt this trust's weight and gift and how it has motivated you to be your best in the dynamic.

Consider the role trust plays in your emotional connection with both the wife and cuckold. How do you demonstrate trust in return? Explore how you can continue to nurture this trust and ensure that it remains the foundation of your relationship moving forward.

Closing Reflection:

Take a deep, grounding breath, and reflect on the meditation, practices, and journaling prompt. Feel gratitude for the trust both the wife and cuckold have given you. Know that this trust is a powerful gift that allows your relationship to grow in strength, respect, and love. As you continue to honor this trust, you are not just fulfilling your role. Still, you are helping to build a foundation of deep emotional connection and mutual respect that benefits everyone involved.

The importance of consent in every encounter

Meditation:

Find a quiet and comfortable space to relax. Close your eyes gently and take a deep breath, filling your lungs with fresh, calming air. As you exhale, let go of any tension or distractions, grounding yourself in the present moment.

Now, focus on the importance of consent in every encounter. Visualize yourself in a situation where respect, communication, and mutual understanding are at the forefront. Whether you're with the wife or the cuckold, your relationship dynamic is built on the foundation of trust, and consent is the cornerstone of that trust.

Picture yourself standing together with both your partner and the cuckold, all three of you in alignment with one another, aware of your needs and desires. You understand that each decision, each action, must be rooted in the respect of everyone's boundaries, desires, and emotional well-being. Consent is not just a one-time agreement—it's an ongoing, dynamic exchange that ensures everyone involved feels heard, valued, and safe.

Visualize asking for and receiving verbal consent in a moment of connection. You ask questions, listen attentively to the responses, and respect the decisions of both partners. Feel the empowerment that comes from clear and open communication. Notice the sense of security it brings, knowing that each interaction is framed with mutual respect and understanding.

As you take another breath, let yourself fully experience the peace from knowing you and your partners are on the same page, making decisions aligned with your shared values and boundaries. With each inhale, breathe in the responsibility and the privilege of practicing consent with care. With each exhale, release doubts or insecurities, knowing that consent is an act of love and trust, not just an obligation.

Affirmation:
"I honor and respect the importance of consent in every encounter. I trust in the process of clear communication, and I empower both my partner and the cuckold to share their desires and boundaries freely."

Practices in Action:

Activity 1: The Consent Check-In

Before engaging in any physical or emotional interaction, please take a moment to check in with both the wife and cuckold about their current comfort levels. Ask them about their boundaries, any changes in desires, or anything new they would like to explore. This is a practice of mindfulness that ensures everyone is aligned and comfortable before moving forward.

Tip: Always be open to hearing "no" or requesting to slow down or pause. Consent is an ongoing dialogue, and it's essential always to remain receptive to each other's needs.

Activity 2: Writing Consent Agreements

Create a written agreement or understanding with your partner and the cuckold that outlines the boundaries, desires, and expectations within your dynamic. This agreement can be revisited, reminding everyone that consent is a living, evolving process. Each person should feel heard and respected, and this written document helps to provide clarity and accountability for everyone involved.

Journaling Prompt:

Reflect on your understanding of consent. How do you ensure that consent is respected in your encounters? When clear and open communication about consent makes you feel empowered and safe. How did it impact the relationship you share with both your partner and the cuckold?

Consider how you can further cultivate a practice of consent in your interactions. What steps can you take to ensure that every encounter is rooted in mutual respect, communication, and understanding? Explore any feelings that arise when you think about consent—what are your values, and how can you express them more fully within your relationships?

Closing Reflection:

Take a deep breath and bring your awareness back to your body. As you reflect on the meditation, practices, and journaling prompt, remember that consent is a gift you give to both yourself and your partners. It creates an environment where everyone feels safe, valued, and respected. Consent is the foundation of love, respect, and connection, and as you continue to practice it, you build a relationship that honors each person's autonomy and desires.

Loving and cherishing the hotwife

Meditation:

Find a comfortable and quiet space where you can relax deeply. Close your eyes and take a slow, deep breath in. Allow your body to release tension with each exhale, grounding yourself in the present moment.

Now, visualize the wife standing before you, not just as a partner in this dynamic but as a woman deserving of love, respect, and admiration. You feel the powerful connection between you, built on trust, mutual understanding, and shared desires.

As you breathe deeply, focus on your love and appreciation for her. You see her not as an object but as a person full of strength, vulnerability, and beauty. You cherish your bond and understand the importance of honoring her desires, boundaries, and independence.

Feel the warmth of affection for her—her courage to embrace her desires, her trust in you, and the vulnerability she allows herself to share. As you acknowledge her, please take a moment to recognize how she empowers herself and the relationship you share. She is the heart of this dynamic, and her joy and fulfillment bring light to all involved.

Visualize yourself holding her in your arms, not possessive or controlling, but in a way that shows your deep love and respect. You cherish her autonomy and choices, knowing she can fully explore and express herself. Her trust in you is a gift; you honor it thoroughly, ensuring she feels seen, heard, and loved.

As you breathe, feel your appreciation for her growing. You are not just involved with her physically; you are invested in her emotional and mental well-being. Your connection is rooted in the joy of seeing her thrive, and you give her the space to be the woman she truly is—strong, confident, and deserving of all the love she desires.

Affirmation:
"I cherish and love the hotwife for who she is—strong, confident, and graceful. I honor her desires and trust, and I am grateful for the deep connection we share."

Practices in Action:

Activity 1: Expressing Appreciation

Please take a moment to write a letter or tell the wife how much you appreciate and cherish her. Acknowledge not just her beauty but her strength, her trust, and the special bond you share. Make sure to highlight how much her autonomy and fulfillment mean to you. Share specific moments when she made you feel deeply connected to her and your relationship.

Tip: Use this exercise to remind yourself of the emotional depth of the relationship, not just the physical aspects. Tell her how much you value her as a person, inside and out.

Activity 2: Active Listening and Validation

Sit down with the wife and listen to her without interruption or judgment. Ask her about her desires, feelings about the dynamic, and anything she needs. Make sure she feels heard and respected. Your role is to validate her experience, whether she is sharing her joys or expressing her needs.

Journaling Prompt:

Reflect on how you show love and respect to the hotwife. How do you ensure she feels physically, emotionally, and mentally cherished? Write about a moment where you expressed deep appreciation for her and explored how it impacted your relationship.

What does it feel like to see the hotwife embrace her desires and explore her autonomy? How can you continue nurturing and supporting her in this journey, ensuring she always feels empowered and loved?

Closing Reflection:

Take a moment to breathe deeply and reflect on the meditation and practices. As you continue your journey with the hotwife, remember that your role is to be her ally, supporter, and greatest admirer. Cherish her desires, honor her boundaries, and appreciate the beautiful bond created when trust, love, and respect are the foundation.

By loving and cherishing her, you empower her and the dynamic, creating a space where all participants can thrive. You are not just her lover in this journey—you are her advocate, her confidant, and her source of support. Let that love continue to guide the relationship forward.

Gratitude for the opportunity to share in the couple's journey

Meditation:

Find a quiet, comfortable place to sit or lie down without distractions. Close your eyes and take a few deep, slow breaths. Inhale deeply, feel the air filling your lungs, and exhale slowly, releasing any tension or stress from your body. Allow your breath to ground you in this moment.

As you begin to relax, think of the couple whose journey you are a part of. Picture them as a unit—two deeply connected people committed to growth, trust, and shared experiences. Visualize yourself as a participant in their journey, not just as an outsider but as someone invited in with respect, confidence, and care.

Please take a moment to acknowledge the honor of being part of their dynamic. Recognize the vulnerability they've shown in opening their hearts and minds to you. This is a physical exchange and an emotional and spiritual connection built on respect and shared values.

Feel gratitude for the opportunity to contribute to their relationship in a way that brings joy, growth, and deeper intimacy. Recognize the importance of your role—not as a replacement, but as someone who helps to enrich their connection. Your presence in their journey is a choice they've made that speaks to their trust in you and your role in their bond.

As you breathe, allow gratitude to fill your heart. Thank the wife for the trust she has placed in you, and thank the cuckold for the love and respect he shows you and his wife. You are a vital part of the dynamic that helps them explore and deepen their connection. With you, this journey is complete.

Imagine the couple's relationship blossoming, supported by the respect and love you bring. Feel the joy of knowing you are a trusted participant in their shared experience, and let this gratitude deepen your connection with both of them.

Affirmation:
"I am deeply grateful for the opportunity to share in this couple's journey. I honor their trust in me and cherish my role in supporting and enhancing their bond."

Practices in Action:

Activity 1: Acknowledging the Couple's Trust

Please take a moment to sit down with the wife and cuckold and express your gratitude for being part of their journey. Tell them you value their trust and the opportunity to contribute to their connection. Acknowledge the importance of your role and the trust they've extended to you in being part of their dynamic.

Tip: Be specific in your gratitude. Reflect on moments when you felt most connected to them and how that connection has enriched your understanding of your role in their relationship.

Activity 2: Supporting the Couple's Growth

Think of one way you can actively support the couple in their journey. This could be through emotional validation, offering thoughtful advice, or simply being present in a way that contributes to their emotional intimacy. Make it a practice to engage with them in a manner that reinforces their bond and shows your commitment to their well-being.

Journaling Prompt:

Reflect on the couple's journey and your role in it. How do you feel being part of their dynamic? What have you learned from the relationship about yourself and relationships in general? Write about a time when you felt incredibly grateful for the connection you shared with them.

What does being trusted by both partners in this journey mean to you? How do you show gratitude for the opportunity to enhance their relationship? Explore the joy and fulfillment that come from contributing to their emotional and relational growth.

Closing Reflection:

Take a moment to breathe deeply and reflect on the meditation and practices. Let gratitude fill your heart as you acknowledge the importance of the journey you share with the couple. As you continue to be part of their story, know that your role is essential to their growth, trust, and love.

Through your contributions—emotional, physical, or supportive—you help them create a deeper connection with one another. This journey concerns pleasure, desire, mutual respect, trust, and commitment to shared growth. As you walk this path, let gratitude guide your every interaction, knowing that your presence in their lives is extraordinary.

Recognizing the power of emotional connection

Meditation:

Sit in a comfortable position, taking a deep breath in, allowing your chest to rise and expand, and slowly exhaling, letting go of any tension in your body. With each breath, feel yourself becoming more present in this moment. Let your mind focus only on your breath, and with every inhale, bring yourself deeper into relaxation.

As you continue to breathe deeply, think about the relationship between the wife and cuckold. Reflect on their emotional bond—how they trust, love, and support each other. Understand that the power of this connection is not just physical but deeply emotional, founded in shared experiences, vulnerability, and mutual respect.

Now, visualize yourself within this dynamic, not as an outsider, but as someone who contributes to this emotional bond. Your presence in their relationship brings physical pleasure and enhances their emotional connection. You are a part of something more significant—something about growth, understanding, and shared joy.

Imagine the depth of the emotional connection between the wife and cuckold as it strengthens through your participation. See how this connection is enriched by respect and trust. Picture the wife feeling loved, empowered, and supported, knowing she is cherished by both you and her husband. Visualize the cuckold finding strength and fulfillment in knowing that his wife's happiness is a reflection of his love and devotion to her.

As you breathe, let this understanding of emotional connection wash over you. Acknowledge how powerful and transformative emotional intimacy can be. It's not only about the physical act; it's about the emotional experiences that create deeper bonds between people. You play a vital role in nurturing these connections and fostering love, trust, and vulnerability.

Affirmation:
"I recognize the power of emotional connection in relationships. I honor the emotional depth I bring to the couple's journey, and I am grateful for the trust and love we share."

Practices in Action:

Activity 1: Emotional Check-In with the Couple

Take some time to connect emotionally with both the wife and cuckold. This could be through a heart-to-heart conversation, where you ask each of them how they feel emotionally in the dynamic. Show genuine interest in their well-being and emotional growth. Reflect on how you can support them not just physically but emotionally as well.

Tip: Emotional connection goes beyond words. Show them that you value their feelings and respect their emotional needs through your actions.

Activity 2: Reflecting on Emotional Fulfillment

Take a moment to journal or reflect on when you felt emotionally connected to the couple. What emotions did you experience? How did your emotional presence affect the dynamic between you all? Consider how this connection has deepened your understanding of intimacy and trust.

Journaling Prompt:

Reflect on the emotional aspects of the relationship you share with the wife and cuckold. How do you recognize and honor their emotional needs? How do you contribute to the emotional intimacy of the dynamic? Write about a specific moment when you felt that emotional connection most profoundly.

What does sharing an emotional connection with your partners mean to you? How does it deepen your respect for both of them and enhance the dynamic between you all? Explore the significance of emotional vulnerability in building a stronger connection.

Closing Reflection:

Breathe deeply and take a moment to feel grateful for the emotional connection you share with the couple. Know that your role is vital to the health and growth of their relationship, and your emotional presence strengthens their bond.

As you continue contributing to their journey, remember that emotional connection is as powerful as physical connection. Your respect, empathy, and understanding make this dynamic fulfilling for everyone involved.

Allow this understanding of emotional depth to guide your interactions, bringing even more closeness, trust, and love into the relationship. Your presence is a gift; through emotional connection, you are helping nurture a bond that will continue to grow and flourish.

Respecting the cuckold's role and emotions

Meditation:

Find a quiet and comfortable space to relax. Please close your eyes, take a deep breath, and let it out slowly. With each breath, feel your body become more relaxed and your mind more focused. Allow any tension or stress to melt away as you bring awareness to the present moment.

Now, bring your thoughts to the cuckold. Picture him standing before you, not as an outsider, but as an essential part of the dynamic—a person whose role is not just physical but deeply emotional and personal. His trust in his partner, vulnerability, and willingness to share his deepest emotions create the foundation for your bond.

As you breathe deeply, reflect on the emotional complexity of his role. Understand that the cuckold's emotions are rooted in love, acceptance, and the courage to embrace his desires, even when they might be challenging to face. His journey is about trust—trust in his partner, you, and yourself.

Visualize him feeling secure in his position, knowing that his value in the relationship is not defined by the physical acts but by the emotional depth and strength of the connection he shares with his wife. Recognize the courage it takes for him to embrace this dynamic entirely and without hesitation. His role is one of emotional strength, support, and love.

See how your presence adds to the cuckold's emotional growth. The respect you show him and the care you communicate and honor his feelings deepen your trust. You contribute to his wife's joy and his sense of emotional fulfillment and self-worth. His role is vital, and your recognition creates a foundation of mutual respect and understanding.

Affirmation:
"I respect the cuckold's role and emotions. I honor his trust, vulnerability, and emotional strength and am grateful for our deep connection."

Practices in Action:

Activity 1: Acknowledging the Cuckold's Emotions

Please take a moment to connect with the cuckold and ask him how he is feeling emotionally. Acknowledge the complexity of his feelings and show empathy for the challenges he may be facing. Recognize the strength it takes for him to be vulnerable in this dynamic. Be open and compassionate in your responses, showing that you value his emotions and role in the relationship.

Tip: Understanding the cuckold's emotions requires patience and openness. Allow him to express his feelings without judgment and offer validation for his role in the dynamic.

Activity 2: Reflecting on His Role

Spend time journaling or reflecting on how you view the cuckold's role in the relationship. How do you see his contributions, both emotional and physical? Write about how you can honor and respect his feelings and explore how you can help create a supportive environment where he feels valued and secure.

Journaling Prompt:

Think about the cuckold's role in this dynamic. How does he contribute to the relationship emotionally? How do his feelings enhance the overall connection between the wife, cuckold, and yourself? Reflect on a time when you felt deeply connected with him emotionally. What emotions did you experience, and how did that deepen your trust?

What can you do to ensure that the cuckold feels fully respected in his role? How can you help him feel supported and valued, not just physically but emotionally and psychologically as well? Write about how you can continue to nurture this emotional respect moving forward.

Closing Reflection:

Take a moment to breathe deeply and reflect on the importance of the cuckold's emotions and role in the dynamic. His vulnerability and trust are foundational to the strength of the relationship, and by respecting and honoring his feelings, you contribute to a deeper emotional connection for everyone involved.

Remember, the cuckold's journey is one of strength, love, and trust. Your ability to recognize and respect his emotional world creates a space for greater connection and fulfillment. As you continue to honor his role, you help create a balanced, nurturing dynamic based on trust, mutual respect, and love.

Creating a harmonious and fulfilling relationship dynamic

Meditation:

Find a calm, comfortable place to settle yourself. Close your eyes, take a deep breath, and release any tension from your body. Let your mind focus solely on the present, setting aside distractions or judgments.

Now, envision the dynamic between yourself, the wife, and the cuckold. Picture it as a beautifully balanced triangle—each side essential, each connection bringing strength and unity. The harmony of this dynamic relies on mutual respect, understanding, and shared purpose.

See yourself within this dynamic, contributing passion, emotional balance, and respect. Recognize the importance of your role—not just as a lover but as part of an intricate connection that uplifts and empowers everyone involved.

Visualize the wife's joy and freedom, the cuckold's pride and support, and your sense of fulfillment as you all share in this unique bond. This harmony is built on trust, honesty, and openness. Honoring each person's needs and emotions helps create an environment where love and understanding thrive.

Reflect on how your presence strengthens the relationship through empathy and mindful action, not by dominance. You are a steward of this connection, contributing to its growth and balance.

Affirmation:
"I honor the harmony of this dynamic. I contribute to a fulfilling and balanced connection through respect, empathy, and mindful action."

Practices in Action:

Activity 1: Open Dialogue Session

Organize a moment with the couple to discuss how the dynamic feels for everyone. Focus on creating an open, judgment-free space where all parties can share their feelings, desires, and boundaries. Listen actively and express your thoughts with respect and honesty.

Tip: Approach this conversation with the intent to understand, not to fix or change. Your role is to foster harmony through clear and empathetic communication.

Activity 2: Practicing Gratitude for the Dynamic

Take time to reflect on what you appreciate about both the wife and the cuckold. Write down three things you value about each person, focusing on their unique contributions to the relationship. Consider sharing these thoughts with them thoughtfully and respectfully to strengthen the bond.

Journaling Prompt:

Reflect on the dynamic you share with the wife and cuckold. What does harmony mean to you in this context? How do you see your role in maintaining balance and ensuring everyone feels respected and valued? Write about a time when the dynamic felt incredibly fulfilling for all parties involved. What contributed to that sense of harmony, and how can you nurture those elements moving forward?

What steps can you take to ensure the relationship dynamic remains respectful, supportive, and fulfilling for everyone? How can you better align your actions with the values of empathy, openness, and shared joy?

Closing Reflection:

Take a deep breath and reflect on the beauty of your connection. The harmony within this dynamic is not accidental; it is cultivated through care, respect, and open communication. By remaining mindful of each person's needs and emotions, you contribute to a bond that is both fulfilling and enduring.

Remember that harmony is built through shared effort and mutual respect as you move forward. You are an essential part of this dynamic, and your actions have the power to nurture love, trust, and understanding.

Embracing the beauty of shared intimacy

Meditation:

Find a quiet place to settle yourself and take a calming breath. Close your eyes and focus on the rhythm of your breathing. Allow the outside world to fade as you bring your attention to the present moment.

Visualize the connection you share with the couple—the trust, openness, and care that make this dynamic possible. Intimacy is more than physical; it's about shared understanding, vulnerability, and emotional resonance. See how your presence within this dynamic brings joy and fulfillment to all involved.

Imagine the moments of closeness you've shared. Feel the depth of connection with the wife as you honor her confidence and freedom. Recognize the strength and selflessness of the cuckold, who finds joy in seeing his partner happy and fulfilled.

This shared intimacy is a gift reflecting trust and mutual respect. It is about moments of passion and creating an environment where everyone feels valued and cherished. You are part of something unique, and your role contributes to the beauty and balance of this relationship.

Breathe in the warmth of connection, and release doubts or hesitations as you exhale. Embrace the beauty of what you share, knowing that your actions are rooted in respect, love, and openness.

Affirmation:
"I honor the intimacy we share, grounded in trust, respect, and mutual fulfillment. This connection reflects love and understanding, and I am grateful for my role."

Practices in Action:

Activity 1: Create a Moment of Appreciation

Plan a gesture of appreciation for the couple. It might be a heartfelt note expressing your gratitude for their trust and openness or a thoughtful action demonstrating your respect for their bond. This small act can deepen the intimacy and understanding you share.

Tip: Acknowledge the emotional depth of the connection rather than the physical aspects. Your sincerity will strengthen the relationship.

Activity 2: Practice Active Listening

During your following conversation with either the wife or the cuckold, dedicate yourself to truly listening. Avoid interrupting or thinking ahead to your response. Please pay attention to their words, emotions, and underlying needs. Active listening fosters emotional intimacy and reinforces trust.

Journaling Prompt:

Reflect on the moments of intimacy you've shared within this dynamic. How does it feel to be trusted and included in such a unique connection? What aspects of shared intimacy do you find most meaningful, and how do they align with your values?

Write about the emotional resonance of these experiences. How have they deepened your understanding of yourself and the couple? What steps can you take to continue fostering a sense of closeness and trust within this relationship?

Closing Reflection:

Take a deep breath, and let your heart be grateful for your shared connection. Shared intimacy is a profound and beautiful bond built on trust, respect, and mutual understanding. By embracing this connection with care and intention, you honor this unique dynamic's emotional and spiritual aspects.

As you move forward, remember that intimacy thrives in an atmosphere of openness and appreciation. Your role is an integral part of this relationship, and by nurturing it, you contribute to something extraordinary.

The joy of seeing both partners satisfied

Meditation:

Close your eyes and take a deep breath, feeling the air fill your lungs. Slowly release the breath, letting go of any tension. As you settle into a calm state, focus on the dynamic you share with the couple—built on trust, respect, and a shared purpose of fulfillment.

Visualize the wife and cuckold together, their bond stronger for the experiences you've shared. Imagine the wife's radiant smile, reflecting her joy and confidence. See the cuckold's contentment, a profound expression of his love and trust in her and you. Recognize the unique role you play in their happiness and unity.

As you reflect, feel a sense of gratitude for being part of something so rare—a relationship dynamic where honesty, respect, and fulfillment intertwine. The joy you witness in both partners is a testament to your cultivated connection. It's not just about moments of pleasure but about nurturing an environment where everyone feels valued and satisfied.

Breathe deeply, embracing the satisfaction of seeing both partners thrive. With each exhale, release doubts, focusing instead on the beauty of the harmony you've helped create.

Affirmation:
"I find joy in seeing both partners fulfilled, knowing that my presence fosters their happiness and strengthens their bond. This dynamic is built on trust, respect, and mutual satisfaction."

Practices in Action:

Activity 1: Acknowledging the Couple's Bond

Take a moment to express your appreciation for the couple's connection. Whether through a thoughtful conversation, a sincere compliment, or a small gesture, acknowledge how their love inspires and informs the dynamic. Celebrating their bond reinforces the trust and respect between you.

Tip: Be genuine and specific. For example, highlight a moment that showed the strength of their relationship or the joy they shared.

Activity 2: Reflecting on Balance

Reflect on how your actions and presence contribute to the couple's happiness. Consider how you can continue to prioritize both partners' feelings and needs in your interactions. This reflection helps ensure your role remains a positive and balanced force in their dynamic.

Journaling Prompt:

Write about a moment when you felt satisfied seeing both partners happy and fulfilled. How did their joy impact you emotionally? What does being part of their journey mean to you, and how do you honor their trust in you?

Explore how you can continue to foster an environment where both partners feel valued. What steps can you take to ensure that your role supports their emotional and relational needs? How does their satisfaction bring meaning and fulfillment to your own experience?

Reflection:

Take a deep breath and feel grateful for your trust and openness with the couple. The joy of seeing both partners satisfied reflects the mutual respect and care that defines your dynamic. You are part of something meaningful and unique, where everyone's happiness is intertwined.

As you move forward, carry this sense of fulfillment with you. By focusing on the well-being and joy of both partners, you create a harmonious and enriching relationship dynamic that celebrates trust, connection and shared satisfaction.

Learning from each experience to grow in love

Meditation:

Find a comfortable position and take a deep breath. Inhale, feeling the moment's fullness, and exhale, releasing distractions. Allow yourself to focus on the journey you've undertaken with the couple. Each experience is a stepping stone in building trust, understanding, and love.

Visualize a path before you, illuminated by the moments you've shared with the couple. Along this path are milestones—conversations that deepened trust, moments of connection that strengthened bonds, and experiences that brought joy and fulfillment to all involved.

See how each moment has shaped you, helping you grow in compassion, empathy, and love. Picture the wife and cuckold walking beside you, each step representing a shared commitment to mutual respect and understanding. Their trust in you has provided a foundation for your growth, just as your role has enriched their journey.

Reflect on your lessons: the importance of clear communication, the beauty of vulnerability, and the value of mutual consent. These lessons are about your role and the more profound principles of love, trust, and respect that guide you.

Breathe deeply, feeling gratitude for the opportunity to grow through these shared experiences. With each exhale, let go of any uncertainties, grounding yourself in the knowledge that each moment, no matter how small, contributes to a more meaningful connection.

Affirmation:
"Every experience is an opportunity to learn and grow in love. I honor the trust given to me and embrace the lessons that deepen our connection."

Practices in Action:

Activity 1: Reflective Growth

Take time after each interaction with the couple to reflect on your learning. Write down a key takeaway—perhaps about communication, understanding their boundaries, or recognizing the dynamics of their relationship. Use these insights to guide your future actions and deepen your connection.

Tip: Approach each experience with curiosity and humility, knowing that growth comes from listening, observing, and reflecting.

Activity 2: Expressing Gratitude for Growth

Please share with the couple how your experiences with them have helped you grow. Whether a simple thank-you or a heartfelt conversation, expressing your gratitude strengthens the bond you share and acknowledges your role in your journey.

Journaling Prompt:

Reflect on a recent experience with the couple. What did you learn about love, trust, or connection? How has this experience shaped your understanding of the dynamic and your role? Write about the emotions that arose and how to use this insight to nurture a deeper connection with both partners.

Think about how your growth impacts the couple. How do your lessons enhance the relationship dynamic? How can you continue to grow as a partner in this journey, contributing to the love and trust you all share?

Closing Reflection:

Breathe deeply and feel gratitude for the growth you've experienced. Each encounter, conversation, and connection has brought you closer to understanding the beauty of love in all its forms. Your lessons guide you in creating more profound, more meaningful relationships.

As you continue this journey, carry these insights with you. Remember that growth is a continuous process, and each moment offers an opportunity to deepen your love, respect, and connection. You are integral to a shared story that thrives on learning and mutual understanding.

Appreciating the love that flows between all of us

Meditation:

Take a deep breath, feeling the air enter your lungs, bringing a sense of calm and connection. Exhale slowly, releasing any tension. Close your eyes and focus on the warmth that flows through you, a love shared and reciprocated among all involved.

Picture yourself in a circle with the wife and cuckold, an unbroken bond of trust, respect, and care connecting you. Feel the energy of love flowing between you, an invisible current that unites and empowers each person in their unique role.

As you visualize this, reflect on the love the wife shares with her husband, the foundation of their bond, and how their openness has allowed you to be part of their journey. Recognize the trust and affection they extend to you, inviting you into their shared experience.

Now, focus inward and notice the love and care you contribute to this dynamic. It is not only about physical connection but emotional understanding and respect. This love flows freely, enhancing and supporting everyone involved. It is a testament to the beauty of connection when trust and openness thrive.

Breathe in this love, letting it fill your heart with gratitude. Breathe out, sending that gratitude back to the couple. Feel the balance between giving and receiving, knowing you are part of something greater—a shared journey of trust, passion, and mutual respect.

Affirmation:
"Love flows freely between us, strengthening our bond. I am grateful for the trust and connection we share, and I honor the beauty of this dynamic."

Practices in Action:

Activity 1: Expressing Gratitude for the Connection

Take a moment to thank both partners for the love and trust they've shown you. Whether through a heartfelt conversation, a written note, or a simple gesture, acknowledging their openness reinforces the strength of your connection.

Tip: Be specific in your gratitude. Highlight moments or actions that have made you feel valued and connected, emphasizing the mutual love and respect you share.

Activity 2: Strengthening the Flow of Love

Plan an activity that allows all three of you to connect emotionally, such as an evening spent sharing stories, laughter, or heartfelt reflections. Focus on creating a space where love and appreciation can flow naturally, strengthening the bond between all participants.

Journaling Prompt:

Reflect on the love that flows between you and the couple. How does this love make you feel connected and valued? Write about how this dynamic has enriched your life and helped you grow emotionally.

Consider the balance of giving and receiving within the relationship. How do you contribute to the flow of love? What can you do to ensure this connection thrives and deepens over time?

Closing Reflection:

Breathe deeply, feeling the love that flows between you and the couple. This bond is a testament to the beauty of shared trust and mutual respect. Carry this feeling of connection with you, knowing you are part of a relationship that values openness, understanding, and care.

As you move forward, honor the love you share and your unique roles in nurturing this bond. Remember, love is not finite—it grows stronger when shared, enriching everyone involved in its embrace.

Feeling the warmth of mutual respect

Meditation:

Sit comfortably and close your eyes. Breathe deeply, allowing the air to flow easily in and out of your body. As you settle into the rhythm of your breath, let your thoughts drift toward the idea of respect—a powerful, grounding force that binds relationships together.

Picture yourself standing with the wife and her husband. Each of you holds a unique place in this dynamic, yet you are equal in your shared commitment to openness and understanding. Imagine a warm light surrounding the three of you, a symbol of mutual respect.

Feel the strength of this respect, rooted in trust, honesty, and shared values. It is the foundation of the connection you all share. Acknowledge the respect the couple has extended to you, welcoming you into their lives and entrusting you with their bond.

Now, reflect on the respect you offer them in return. This respect is expressed through listening, honoring boundaries, and cherishing their trust in you. It nurtures the connection, allowing it to flourish and grow stronger.

Breathe in this warmth, this sense of mutual respect, and let it fill your heart. Exhale slowly, sending gratitude and love back to them. In this shared space of respect, you find harmony, understanding, and deep connection.

Affirmation:
"I honor the respect we share and cherish the connection it nurtures. Through mutual understanding, we grow together in trust and love."

Practices in Action:

Activity 1: Acknowledging Respect in Words

Please take a moment to express your respect to the wife and her husband. Share how their openness and trust have impacted you, and let them know how much you value the dynamic you share.

Tip: Approach this conversation with sincerity and mindfulness. Let your words reflect your genuine appreciation and care.

Activity 2: Practicing Respectful Listening

The next time you're with the couple, practice active listening. Whether they share their thoughts, desires, or boundaries, focus entirely on their words without interrupting or anticipating your response. Show them that their voices are heard and valued.

Journaling Prompt:

Reflect on how mutual respect affects your connection with the couple. How do you feel when you receive their respect, and how do you show them respect in return?

Write about a moment where you felt the warmth of this mutual respect. How did it strengthen your bond? Consider how you can continue to nurture this foundation as your relationship evolves.

Closing Reflection:

Take a deep breath and feel the grounding presence of mutual respect. It is a force that enriches your connection and fosters more profound understanding and trust.

As you move forward, carry this respect in all your interactions, letting it guide your words and actions. Remember, respect is the cornerstone of meaningful relationships; love and connection thrive through it.

Trust and loyalty in my relationships

Meditation:

Find a quiet space where you can sit comfortably. Close your eyes and take a deep, calming breath. Let the air fill your lungs, and as you exhale, imagine releasing any doubts or uncertainties.

Picture yourself standing in a bond built on trust and loyalty. See the wife and her husband before you, offering their trust openly. This trust is not given lightly; it is a gift earned through respect, honesty, and consistent care.

Reflect on how loyalty manifests in your actions. It is how you honor their boundaries, respect their relationship, and prioritize open communication. Imagine these actions weaving a robust and golden thread that connects you to them—a thread of unwavering trust.

Feel the warmth of their loyalty in return. They have chosen to share this dynamic with you, and in doing so, they offer a piece of themselves. This mutual loyalty creates a safe, supportive space where everyone can thrive and feel valued.

Breathe deeply into this moment, letting the feelings of trust and loyalty fill your heart. With each exhale, release any lingering fears or insecurities, knowing this bond is built on mutual care and respect.

Affirmation:
"I nurture trust and loyalty in my relationships, creating a bond that strengthens and uplifts us all."

Practices in Action:

Activity 1: Reaffirming Trust Through Communication

Take time to have an open conversation with the wife and her husband. Reaffirm your commitment to respecting their boundaries and nurturing the trust you share. Share one way you've seen trust grow in your relationship and ask them how to continue to honor that bond.

Tip: Approach this conversation with humility and genuine curiosity. Listening is just as essential as speaking in building trust.

Activity 2: Showing Loyalty in Action

Think of one thoughtful gesture you can offer to demonstrate your loyalty to both partners. It might be as simple as checking in to see how they feel or expressing gratitude for their trust. Actions that align with their needs reinforce your shared connection.

Journaling Prompt:

Reflect on how trust and loyalty shape your connection with the couple. In what ways have they shown their trust in you, and how have you shown loyalty to them?

Consider a time when trust deepened your bond. How did that moment make you feel? What did it teach you about the importance of loyalty in your relationships? Write about ways to continue building on this foundation of trust and loyalty.

Closing Reflection:

As you finish, take a deep breath and feel the strength of trust and loyalty in your relationships. These qualities are the bedrock of meaningful connections, providing a safe space where love and respect flourish.

Carry this understanding with you as you move forward. Trust is nurtured by honesty and care, and loyalty is shown through consistent, thoughtful actions. Together, they create a bond that uplifts and sustains everyone involved.

Opening my heart to deep emotional connections

Meditation:

Find a quiet place to sit and relax. Take a deep breath, feeling the air expand within you, and then exhale slowly, releasing any tension. Close your eyes and let your mind settle into a calm, reflective state.

Picture yourself in a space of safety and warmth. Surrounding you are the wife and her husband, both radiating acceptance and trust. This space is free of judgment, a sanctuary where authentic emotional connections can thrive.

Focus on your heart. Imagine it as a door that you gently open, inviting vulnerability and genuine connection. See the moments you've shared with the couple, not just in passion but in shared smiles, conversations, and mutual respect. Each moment has strengthened your bond, creating an emotional depth beyond the surface.

Feel the courage to open your heart fully—to be honest, present, and emotionally available. As you breathe deeply, imagine this connection growing stronger, rooted in trust and mutual care. With each breath, allow gratitude to fill your heart for the opportunity to form such meaningful bonds.

You are not merely a participant in this dynamic but a valued and respected part of their lives. Let this truth ground you as you nurture these emotional connections with openness and sincerity.

Affirmation:
"I open my heart to deep emotional connections, embracing vulnerability and trust as pathways to love and understanding."

Practices in Action:

Activity 1: Sharing from the Heart

Set aside time to have a heartfelt conversation with the wife or husband. Share something meaningful about your feelings in this dynamic, focusing on the emotional bond you've built. Invite them to share their feelings, creating a moment of mutual vulnerability.

Tip: Approach this conversation with sincerity and mindfulness. Active listening and validation of their emotions will deepen the connection further.

Activity 2: Reflective Letter Writing

Write a letter to the couple expressing gratitude for your shared emotional depth. Include specific moments that have strengthened your bond and how these connections have enriched your life. Even if you don't share the letter, writing will help you recognize and appreciate the emotional intimacy you've cultivated.

Journaling Prompt:

Think about the emotional connections you've formed with the couple. What does it feel like to open your heart and be vulnerable with them? How have these deep connections enriched your life?

Reflect on a time when emotional intimacy felt especially strong. What was it about that moment that made it so impactful? How can you foster openness and trust in your relationships moving forward?

Closing Reflection:

As you finish this meditation, take a moment to appreciate the courage it takes to open your heart to others. Deep emotional connections are built on trust, vulnerability, and mutual respect, which you actively nurture in your relationships.

Carry this sense of openness with you. Remember, by embracing emotional depth, you are creating a space where love and understanding can flourish, enriching your life and the lives of those you connect with.

Feeling the power of positive energy in shared moments

Meditation:

Close your eyes and take a deep, calming breath. Let the air fill your lungs, and as you exhale, release any tension in your shoulders, neck, and chest. Feel your body relax as you tune into the present moment.

Picture yourself in the company of the couple—two people who have welcomed you into their lives with trust and openness. Focus on the shared moments you've experienced, filled with warmth, laughter, and connection. Visualize these moments as glowing orbs of light surrounding you, each representing the positive energy you've exchanged.

Feel the energy from these shared experiences flow through you like a warm current, uplifting and renewing your spirit. Each moment you've shared has contributed to a deeper bond, a greater understanding, and mutual joy.

As you sit with this feeling, acknowledge your role in creating and amplifying this energy. Your presence, sincerity, and respect help foster an environment where everyone can feel valued and fulfilled.

Breathe deeply, allowing this positive energy to expand within you. Imagine bringing this light forward, bringing more joy and connection to your shared experiences.

Affirmation:
"I embrace the positive energy in shared moments, knowing that my presence contributes to joy, trust, and connection."

Practices in Action:

Activity 1: Reflect on Shared Joy

Reflect on a moment that brought joy to all three of you. Please write it down or share it with the couple, expressing gratitude for the positive energy you felt at that moment. Let them know how it impacted you emotionally.

Tip: Be specific when recalling the moment—whether it was a shared laugh, an open conversation, or a kind gesture. This will deepen the connection and appreciation.

Activity 2: Creating a Joyful Memory

Plan an activity or gesture that celebrates your bond, such as sharing a meal, walking, or engaging in meaningful conversation. Focus on being fully present, and notice how the energy shifts as you connect with them on a deeper level.

Journaling Prompt:

Reflect on a shared moment that filled you with positive energy. What made it so memorable? How did you feel about yourself and your connection with the couple?

Explore how you can continue to create and nurture these moments of positivity. What role do you play in bringing joy and energy to your shared experiences?

Closing Reflection:

As you finish this meditation, take a deep breath and smile, feeling the warmth of positive energy. Each shared moment is a gift—an opportunity to connect, uplift, and strengthen your bond.

Carry this awareness with you as you move forward. By embracing the power of positive energy, you contribute to an environment where joy, love, and mutual respect thrive.

Celebrating the bond that transcends traditional labels

Meditation:

Find a quiet space and settle into a comfortable position. Close your eyes and take a deep, grounding breath. As you inhale, imagine drawing in acceptance and love. As you exhale, relinquish any judgments or preconceived notions about roles or labels.

Visualize the connection you share with the couple. Conventional definitions or societal expectations do not confine it. Instead, it's a bond rooted in authenticity, trust, and mutual respect. See the three of you standing together, each contributing your unique presence to create something extraordinary—a relationship that transcends boundaries and limitations.

Feel the strength of this bond, the way it allows each of you to express your true selves. There is no hierarchy here, only a shared purpose: to uplift one another and find joy in your connection.

As you consider this vision, express gratitude for the opportunity to be part of something so profound. Celebrate the freedom of embracing this dynamic and the beauty of the love and respect that flows between you.

Take a few more breaths, holding onto the warmth and appreciation for this bond. When you're ready, open your eyes and carry this sense of celebration with you.

Affirmation:
"I honor and celebrate the bond we share, knowing it transcends traditional labels and thrives on trust, respect, and authenticity."

Practices in Action:

Activity 1: Acknowledging the Unique Connection

Take time to express gratitude to the couple for the dynamic you share. Write or say something that acknowledges the uniqueness of your bond, emphasizing how much you appreciate the trust and authenticity that define your relationship.

Tip: Focus on how this connection allows everyone involved to grow and feel fulfilled rather than on specific roles or labels.

Activity 2: Create a Symbol of Your Bond

Collaborate with the couple to create a small, symbolic gesture representing your unique connection. It could be a shared keepsake, a meaningful phrase, or even a shared memory you consciously create together. Let this symbol serve as a reminder of the bond that transcends definitions.

Journaling Prompt:

Reflect on how this dynamic allows you to connect with others in a way that feels genuine and free of societal expectations. How does this bond challenge or redefine traditional ideas of relationships for you?

Write about what it feels like to be part of a relationship built on trust and respect rather than rigid roles. How has it helped you grow as an individual and as a participant in this dynamic?

Closing Reflection:

As you reflect on this meditation, take a moment to appreciate the uniqueness of your bond. It is a rare and beautiful connection, defined not by labels but by the love, trust, and joy that unite you.

Carry this awareness into your daily life, knowing that by honoring and celebrating this bond, you contribute to something extraordinary and transformative.

THE CUCKOLD

Welcome to the cuckold's journey, where love, trust, and emotional growth intertwine to create a dynamic that is deeply fulfilling and transformative. In this space, you will explore your unique role with pride, acceptance, and understanding, finding joy in your partner's happiness and fulfillment. This journey is one of profound emotional connection, where the love and respect shared between you and your wife are the foundation for a bond that continues to evolve.

In the cuckold dynamic, your strength comes not from dominance but from your unwavering support, trust, and the deep emotional connection you share. You have a vital role in your relationship, which is built on mutual respect, communication, and the understanding that your fulfillment is tied to your partner's happiness. Here, you will find the space to appreciate your wife's desires and joys and the opportunity to grow emotionally, deepening the connection that binds you together.

Each meditation, affirmation, and practice will guide you in honoring your feelings of love, admiration, and gratitude while empowering you to embrace your role with openness and pride. You will learn to recognize the strength of vulnerability, the joy from seeing your partner thrive, and the beauty of a relationship founded on trust, mutual respect, and shared love.

You will gain clarity, insight, and emotional fulfillment through this journey. You will experience the deep satisfaction of loving with an open heart, nurturing your growth, and celebrating the joy that blossoms between you, your wife, and the beautiful dynamic you create together.

Embracing my role with pride

Meditation:

Sit comfortably in a quiet place and take a deep breath. Let the air fill your lungs, and as you exhale, release any tension or doubt you may be holding. Close your eyes and bring your focus to your heart.

Visualize yourself in your chosen role, filled with love, trust, and understanding. See your wife standing before you, radiant with confidence and joy. She looks at you with deep affection and appreciation. Know that your willingness to embrace this dynamic is a gift—a demonstration of your love, strength, and commitment to her happiness.

As you reflect on this, allow feelings of inadequacy or societal judgment to fade. See them dissipate like clouds in the sky. In their place, let pride and self-respect fill you. You have chosen this path out of love, and that love strengthens the bond between you and your wife.

Feel your heart open to the joy of seeing her fulfilled, to the connection that grows from your shared honesty and vulnerability. You are not defined by what others think; the love determines you and the trust you nurture within your relationship.

Breathe in deeply, feeling this pride and love anchor you. With each breath, affirm your role is one of strength and devotion. When ready, open your eyes, holding onto this pride and purpose.

Affirmation:
"I embrace my role with pride and love, knowing it strengthens my connection with my wife and deepens our trust."

Practices in Action:

Activity 1: Celebrate Your Unique Bond

Write your wife a heartfelt letter expressing why you value your role in the relationship. Share how it deepens your love for her and strengthens your trust. Please focus on your pride in contributing to her happiness and fulfillment.

Tip: Be honest and vulnerable, letting her know how this dynamic brings you joy and satisfaction, even in moments of challenge.

Activity 2: Engage in a Moment of Reflection

Reflect on how embracing your role has positively impacted your relationship. Write down three ways this dynamic has brought you closer to your wife and how it has helped you grow as a person.

Journaling Prompt:

Reflect on what embracing your role with pride means to you. How does it change the way you view yourself and your relationship? What moments did you feel deep fulfillment in this dynamic, and how can you carry that feeling forward?

Write about the strength and love you feel in choosing this role. How has it challenged or inspired you to grow emotionally, and how does it reflect the depth of your commitment to your wife?

Closing Reflection:

Take a moment to honor yourself for the love, courage, and pride you bring to this relationship. By embracing your role with an open heart, you strengthen the bond between you and your wife and build trust and mutual understanding.

Carry this pride with you, knowing that your role is a powerful expression of love and a testament to the strength of your connection.

The joy of seeing my partner fulfilled

Meditation:

Find a comfortable position and close your eyes. Take a deep breath, feel the air fill your lungs, and exhale slowly, releasing tension. As you breathe deeply, let your mind settle into a calm and open state.

Visualize your partner, your wife, radiating happiness and confidence. See the glow in her eyes, the smile on her face, and the joy she carries within herself. Feel the warmth of her energy, knowing that her happiness reflects the love and trust you share.

Now, imagine yourself present and supportive in this moment. Let the feelings of pride and joy wash over you as you witness her experiencing fulfillment in her life and desires. Your love creates a space where she can be herself fully, without hesitation or fear.

Reflect on how this dynamic strengthens your bond and deepens your connection. Recognize the courage and love it takes to prioritize her happiness and how it enriches your life. As you hold this image, feel gratitude for the trust and openness that defines your relationship.

Breathe deeply, letting the joy of her fulfillment settle in your heart. When you are ready, open your eyes, carrying this sense of pride and connection with you.

Affirmation:
"I find joy and pride in seeing my partner fulfilled, knowing it strengthens our bond and reflects our love."

Practices in Action:

Activity 1: Create a Moment of Celebration

Plan a special evening to celebrate your wife and the joy she brings to your life. Focus on her achievements, passions, or moments that have fulfilled her. Share with her how proud you are of her and how her happiness positively affects your relationship.

Tip: This celebration doesn't need to be elaborate—the intention matters. A heartfelt conversation or a handwritten note can be as meaningful as a grand gesture.

Activity 2: Reflect on Fulfillment

Set aside time to journal or meditate on how your partner's happiness enhances your own. Write down three ways her fulfillment has positively impacted your emotional connection, relationship role, and personal growth.

Journaling Prompt:

How does seeing your wife fulfilled bring you joy? Reflect on moments when her happiness has deepened your bond and clarified your role in the relationship.

Write about the connection between her fulfillment and your sense of purpose. How does this dynamic reflect the love and trust you share? How can you continue nurturing her happiness while honoring your emotions and needs?

Closing Reflection:

Take a moment to honor the beauty of your relationship. By supporting your wife's fulfillment, you enhance her life and build a stronger, more loving bond between you.

Carry this reflection with you, knowing that the joy you find in her happiness is a powerful testament to the depth of your love and the strength of your partnership.

Building strength through trust

Meditation:

Sit comfortably, close your eyes, and take a calming breath. Let your body relax as you exhale, releasing any tension. Focus on your breathing, letting it guide you to a place of stillness and openness.

Visualize your relationship as a sturdy bridge connecting you and your wife. Each plank of this bridge represents an act of trust—moments where you've shared your deepest thoughts, expressed your desires, or supported one another.

Picture yourself walking across this bridge, step by step, feeling its strength beneath your feet. Reflect on how your trust allows this connection to withstand challenges, grow more robust, and support both of you.

Now imagine your wife standing on the other side of the bridge, smiling warmly at you. Feel her trust in you, just as you trust in her. This mutual belief in one another is the foundation of your dynamic, allowing you both to explore and grow without fear.

As you breathe in, let the strength of this trust fill you, empowering your role in the relationship. With each exhale, release any doubts or insecurities. Trust is your anchor, your guide, and your strength.

Open your eyes and carry this sense of resilience and connection when ready.

Affirmation:
"Trust is the foundation of our relationship, building strength and deepening our connection with each shared moment."

Practices in Action:

Activity 1: Strengthen Your Trust Bridge

Take time to have an open, honest conversation with your wife. Share something personal—a thought, a dream, or a feeling you've been holding onto. Allow her to do the same. This exchange reinforces the trust that keeps your connection strong.

Tip: Approach this conversation with vulnerability and without judgment. Trust is built when both partners feel safe to share their truths.

Activity 2: Create a Symbol of Trust

Work together to create a physical or symbolic representation of your trust—a keepsake, a written promise, or even a shared ritual. Let this symbol serve as a reminder of the strength of your bond and the trust you both nurture.

Journaling Prompt:

Reflect on the role of trust in your relationship. What moments have shown you the strength of the bond you share? How has trust empowered you in your role and deepened your connection with your wife?

Consider times when trust has been tested and how you overcame those challenges together. Write about how you can continue to build trust and strengthen your relationship moving forward.

Closing Reflection:

Trust is the cornerstone of any meaningful relationship and holds an even greater power in your dynamic. By embracing trust, you build strength and a connection that transcends expectations.

Carry this reflection forward, knowing that each act of trust you share fortifies the bond between you and your wife, allowing your relationship to flourish in love and respect.

Recognizing my unique love for her

Meditation:

Find a quiet place where you feel safe and at peace. Sit comfortably, close your eyes, and take a slow, deep breath. As you exhale, let go of any distractions or doubts. Allow yourself to focus entirely on the love you feel for your wife.

Picture her in your mind, smiling and radiating joy. Let yourself feel the depth of your emotions—love, admiration, and pride. This love is yours, unique and unwavering, built on shared experiences, mutual understanding, and deep trust.

Reflect on the ways your love for her is expressed in this relationship. It is not confined by convention but expansive, allowing her to pursue her desires while cherishing your bond. Feel the joy that comes from supporting her and witnessing her happiness.

Now imagine holding her hands, looking into her eyes, and saying, "I love you for all you are." Let this sentiment fill your heart. This love is your strength, your foundation, and your guide. It is a love that adapts, grows, and honors her fully.

With each breath, affirm your commitment to this love. Recognize that it is yours and enough. When ready, open your eyes, carrying this sense of pride and fulfillment.

Affirmation:
"My love for her is unique, boundless, and unwavering. Seeing her thrive and happy to support her desires brings joy."

Practices in Action:

Activity 1: Write a Love Letter

Write a heartfelt letter to your wife, expressing your love and admiration for her. Share specific moments that have strengthened your bond and explain how this dynamic has deepened your connection. Let the letter serve as a tangible reminder of your unique love for her.

Tip: Focus on the emotional aspects of your love, emphasizing your pride in her and your appreciation for the life you've built together.

Activity 2: Celebrate Her Joy

Plan a small surprise or gesture to celebrate her. It could be as simple as preparing her favorite meal, creating a playlist of songs that remind you of her, or organizing a thoughtful date. Show her that your love is expressed in words and meaningful actions.

Journaling Prompt:

Reflect on the unique aspects of your love for your wife. What sets it apart from traditional expressions of love? How does this dynamic deepen your connection and bring you both joy?

Consider the moments when you've felt most proud of her and how supporting her has enriched your relationship. Write about how you can continue to honor and nurture this love in ways that celebrate her individuality and your shared bond.

Closing Reflection:

Love is an ever-evolving journey, and your love with your wife is a testament to the beauty of individuality and connection. It is a unique bond that thrives on openness, respect, and shared joy.

Carry this awareness with you, knowing your love is a gift—a deeply personal and transformative force that uplifts and strengthens both of you.

Feeling gratitude for the freedom to experience her happiness

Meditation:

Find a comfortable, quiet space where you can relax fully. Please close your eyes and take a deep breath, holding it for a moment before slowly exhaling. As you do, imagine releasing any tension or worry, creating room for peace and gratitude.

Visualize your wife in a moment of pure joy, her happiness radiating like sunlight. See her smiling, confident, and fulfilled. Allow yourself to truly bask in this image of her contentment, knowing that your support and love have helped create this space for her.

Focus on the freedom this dynamic has brought into your relationship—the freedom for her to express herself fully and for you to share in her journey. Embrace the realization that her joy enhances your connection and strengthens your love.

Breathe deeply and reflect on the trust and openness you have cultivated together. Feel gratitude for the unique bond that allows you to witness and celebrate her happiness with each exhale. It is a gift to love someone so deeply, see them thrive and grow, and know their joy is yours.

When ready, open your eyes, carrying this sense of gratitude and fulfillment into your day.

Affirmation:
"I am grateful for the freedom to support and celebrate her happiness, knowing that her joy enriches our bond and strengthens our love."

Practices in Action:

Activity 1: Celebrate Together

Please take a moment to celebrate her happiness intentionally. Plan an activity that allows you to express your pride in her—whether it's a heartfelt conversation, a special dinner, or a simple gesture that shows her how much you cherish her joy.

Tip: Let her know how her happiness makes you feel, focusing on the emotional connection it brings to your relationship.

Activity 2: Gratitude Journal

Start a gratitude journal specifically for your relationship. Each day, write down one thing you're grateful for about your dynamic and one way her happiness has inspired or fulfilled you. Over time, this will become a powerful reminder of the beauty in your connection.

Journaling Prompt:

Reflect on what it means to see your wife happy and fulfilled. How does her joy impact your feelings of love and connection? Write about your gratitude for the freedom to experience her happiness and how it enriches your life together.

Consider how this dynamic has brought you closer as a couple and how her happiness allows you to grow and evolve within your role. What steps can you take to continue fostering this gratitude and love?

Closing Reflection:

Gratitude is a cornerstone of love, and through this unique journey, you've found a way to celebrate her happiness and the profound connection it brings to your relationship.

Carry this gratitude with you, knowing that every joy she experiences reflects your love and trust. You are part of something extraordinary, a bond that transcends boundaries and grows through mutual understanding and care.

Experiencing joy in her satisfaction

Meditation:

Find a calm and comfortable place to settle your thoughts. Please close your eyes and take a deep breath, holding it for a moment before exhaling slowly. With each breath, let go of tension, creating space in your heart for peace and joy.

Visualize your wife as happiest, her face lit with satisfaction and fulfillment. Imagine this moment not as something separate from you but as a shared experience that deepens your connection. Her joy is your joy, a testament to the love and trust you both nurture.

Please focus on the energy of her satisfaction, radiating outward and enveloping you both. Feel how this dynamic strengthens your bond, allowing her to flourish while reinforcing your confidence in the relationship.

Breathe in deeply, letting the warmth of her happiness fill your heart. As you exhale, release doubts or fears, replacing them with pride and contentment. Her satisfaction is a reflection of your support, your love, and your shared journey.

When you are ready, please open your eyes, carrying with you the knowledge that her joy celebrates your unique connection.

Affirmation:
"I enjoy her satisfaction, knowing that her happiness strengthens our bond and reflects our love."

Practices in Action:

Activity 1: Share in Her Joy

When your wife shares a moment of satisfaction or fulfillment, take the time to listen and celebrate with her actively. Ask her how the experience made her feel, and express your pride in her.

Tip: Use this moment to strengthen your connection by affirming her desires and the mutual trust you've built together.

Activity 2: Reflective Appreciation

Set aside time to reflect on moments when you've seen her at her happiest. Write down how those moments made you feel and why they were significant. Share these reflections with her to deepen your emotional connection.

Journaling Prompt:

Reflect on a moment when you felt immense joy seeing her happy and satisfied. How did that moment strengthen your love and deepen your understanding of your role in the relationship?

Explore the emotions that arose in you during that time. What aspects of her satisfaction brought you the most joy, and how can you nurture that sense of fulfillment?

Closing Reflection:

Your ability to find joy in her satisfaction is a testament to the depth of your love and the strength of your bond. Celebrating her happiness reinforces the foundation of trust and openness that sustains your connection.

Carry this understanding with you, embracing each moment of her joy as a shared triumph of love, care, and mutual respect. Together, you create a dynamic that is as unique as it is fulfilling.

Strengthening our bond through openness

Meditation:

Find a quiet space where you can relax without interruptions. Close your eyes and take a deep, calming breath. With each inhale, invite peace and clarity into your mind. With each exhale, release any lingering tension or fear.

Picture a bridge connecting you and your wife, built on honesty, trust, and love. This strong bridge grows even sturdier with each moment of openness you share. Visualize yourself walking across this bridge, meeting her halfway, where both of you stand as equals, ready to share your thoughts, feelings, and desires.

Feel the strength of your bond as you open your heart to her. Imagine her doing the same, creating a cycle of understanding and trust. This openness doesn't weaken you; it fortifies your connection, deepening the love and respect you share.

As you focus on this image, reflect on how openness has brought you closer in the past and will continue to do so. Breathe deeply, filling your heart with courage and confidence in your role. Breathe out any hesitation, replacing it with peace and gratitude.

When you're ready, open your eyes, feeling renewed in your commitment to fostering openness and trust in your relationship.

Affirmation:
"I strengthen our bond through honesty and openness, knowing it deepens our love and trust."

Practices in Action:

Activity 1: Initiate a Heartfelt Conversation

Find a time when you and your wife can sit together without distractions. Share one thought or feeling you've been holding onto, and invite her to do the same. Embrace this moment as a chance to deepen your connection.

Tip: Approach the conversation with curiosity and love. Focus on listening to understand rather than responding.

Activity 2: Create an Openness Ritual

Establish a regular time to discuss your feelings and experiences within your dynamic. Use this time to express appreciation for each other and discuss any desires or boundaries. Let this practice become a cornerstone of your relationship.

Journaling Prompt:

Reflect on a time when openness brought you closer to your wife. How did that experience make you feel, and what did you learn about her, yourself, and your relationship?

Write about the importance of vulnerability in your dynamic. How can you embrace openness to strengthen your bond and ensure mutual fulfillment? What steps can you take to cultivate this openness more consistently?

Closing Reflection:

Openness is the key to nurturing trust, love, and understanding in your relationship. Each honest conversation and shared moment of vulnerability brings you closer together, reinforcing your unique bond.

As you continue your journey, remember that openness is not a risk—it's a gift. By embracing it, you create a safe and loving space where your connection can flourish and deepen.

The beauty of vulnerability and trust

Meditation:

Find a comfortable position, either seated or lying down. Close your eyes and breathe deeply through your nose, feeling your chest rise. Exhale slowly through your mouth, releasing any tension or doubts. Repeat this a few times, allowing yourself to relax fully.

Picture a delicate but unbreakable thread connecting you to your wife. This thread is built from moments of honesty, trust, and shared vulnerability. Each time you open your heart to her, the thread strengthens, shimmering with the light of your bond.

Now, recall a moment when you allowed yourself to be genuinely vulnerable—when you shared your deepest feelings or fears and were met with love and acceptance. Let that memory fill you with warmth, reminding you of the strength to be open.

Feel the trust that flows between you, a trust that empowers both of you to explore this unique connection. It's not weakness but courage that lets you share yourself so completely. Embrace this truth: vulnerability is not something to fear but to honor, as it creates a foundation of love and understanding.

Take one more deep breath in, feeling your chest fill with gratitude for the trust you've built. As you exhale, imagine your bond growing even more vital, glowing with mutual respect and love.

Affirmation:
"I embrace the beauty of vulnerability and trust, knowing it deepens my love and strengthens our bond."

Practices in Action:

Activity 1: Share a Vulnerable Thought

Think of something you've been hesitant to share with your wife, whether it's a feeling, a desire, or a fear. Choose a quiet moment to open up to her. Frame your words with love and trust, and invite her to share something in return.

Tip: If you feel nervous, start with something small. The goal is to create a space where vulnerability feels safe and natural.

Activity 2: A Trust-Building Exercise

Set aside time to reflect together on the trust you've built. Share specific instances when her words or actions made you feel safe and valued. Then, discuss how you can continue to nurture this trust.

Journaling Prompt:

Write about a time when being vulnerable in your relationship strengthened your bond. How did it feel to open up, and how did your wife respond?

Explore how trust and vulnerability enhance your dynamic. What steps can you take to foster these qualities in your connection? What might you need to let go of to embrace vulnerability more fully?

Closing Reflection:

Vulnerability and trust are the cornerstones of a deep and meaningful relationship. Allowing yourself to be seen as you are allows love and acceptance to flourish.

Each moment of trust you share strengthens your connection's foundation, allowing you and your wife to grow closer in love and understanding. As you move forward, carry the knowledge that your courage to be vulnerable is a gift that enriches your bond.

Loving with acceptance and an open heart

Meditation:

Settle into a quiet space where you can be comfortable and undisturbed. Close your eyes and take a deep, calming breath through your nose. Hold it gently for a moment, and then release it slowly through your mouth. With each breath, let go of any tension, doubt, or fear and invite peace to fill your heart.

Picture your wife standing before you, her smile radiant and energy full of joy. See her as the incredible person she is—unique, vibrant, and accessible. Notice how her happiness uplifts you and creates a ripple of love that fills the space between you.

Now, imagine opening your heart completely, as if throwing the doors of a beautiful home wide. See love, acceptance, and gratitude pouring out to meet her. There is no judgment, no hesitation—only the pure intention to celebrate her for all she is.

Feel the strength in your love, a love that does not seek to possess but to honor, cherish, and nurture. You are not just a spectator in her happiness but an integral part of it, supporting and amplifying her joy with your acceptance.

Breathe deeply, and as you exhale, let the warmth of this connection fill you. Know that loving with an open heart creates a space where trust and intimacy flourish.

Affirmation:
"I love with acceptance and an open heart, embracing the joy and freedom that strengthens our bond."

Practices in Action:

Activity 1: A Moment of Appreciation

Take time to write a letter to your wife expressing what you love and admire most about her. Focus on her individuality, her passions, and the joy she brings to your life. Please share this letter with her during a quiet, intimate moment.

Tip: Use this to celebrate her without expecting anything in return. The act of giving love unconditionally strengthens your bond.

Activity 2: Practicing Heart-Opening Visualization

Each day, spend five minutes visualizing your love flowing openly and freely toward your wife. Imagine this love surrounding her warmly, bringing her comfort and joy. Reflect on how this practice strengthens your connection.

Journaling Prompt:

How does it feel to love with acceptance and an open heart? Write about moments when you've embraced your wife's happiness wholeheartedly.

Reflect on the ways this dynamic has deepened your connection. Are there areas where you could let go of control or fear to love more freely? How can you continue to show her acceptance and encouragement?

Closing Reflection:

Loving with acceptance and an open heart is a courageous act of devotion. It requires trust, vulnerability, and a commitment to celebrating your partner for who they are.

As you practice this kind of love, you'll find it strengthens your relationship and enriches your sense of self. The openness you share creates a space where you and your wife can thrive, united by the depth of your connection.

Celebrating the love we share in all its forms

Meditation:

Find a peaceful spot to relax and settle your thoughts. Please close your eyes and take a deep breath, holding it for a moment and then exhaling slowly. Feel yourself grounded in the present moment, where love and gratitude dwell.

Picture your relationship as a tapestry, each thread representing a different kind of love: romantic, emotional, physical, and spiritual. Notice how each thread is unique yet woven together, creating something beautiful, substantial, and one-of-a-kind.

Focus on your wife, the central figure in this tapestry. Visualize her laughter, smile, and joy. See how her happiness adds vibrant colors to the fabric of your shared love. Then, picture yourself beside her, your presence steady and supportive, adding depth and warmth to this intricate creation.

Acknowledge that love can take many forms, each equally valid and precious in your relationship. The romantic moments, the shared laughter, the vulnerable conversations, and even the passion you both find in unique ways contribute to the rich, multifaceted bond you share.

As you breathe deeply, embrace the truth that your love is expansive, resilient, and ever-growing. It transcends traditional definitions, existing purely in its authenticity and strength. Celebrate the beauty of what you and your wife have created together.

Affirmation:
"I celebrate the love we share in all forms, embracing the unique bond that unites us."

Practices in Action:

Activity 1: A Day of Celebration

Plan a day dedicated to celebrating your relationship. Choose activities highlighting the different forms of love you share—perhaps a romantic dinner, a hobby, or a meaningful conversation. Reflect together on your journey and the joys you've experienced.

Tip: Focus on being present in each moment, appreciating the love that flows between you in all its beautiful forms.

Activity 2: Love in Writing

Write a list of the ways your love manifests in your relationship. Be as specific as possible, noting the small, everyday moments and the larger, more profound ones. Please share this list with your wife and invite her to add her thoughts.

Journaling Prompt:

Reflect on the different forms of love in your relationship. How does your bond with your wife go beyond traditional expectations? What are the unique ways you show love to one another, and how do these expressions deepen your connection?

Write about a moment when you felt incredibly grateful for the love you share. What made it meaningful, and how can you celebrate that kind of love more often?

Closing Reflection:

Love is as infinite as it is profound, revealing itself in many forms throughout a relationship. Celebrating each of these expressions strengthens the foundation of your bond and creates space for an even more significant connection.

Take a moment to honor the unique love you and your wife share, a love that defies convention yet remains steadfast in its truth. Know that every form of love you experience together is a gift, and every celebration enriches your life's tapestry.

The power of mutual respect in our relationship

Meditation:

Sit in a comfortable position and take a deep breath. Let each inhale fill you with peace, and each exhale release any tension. As you focus on your breath, focus on the concept of respect—the bedrock upon which all strong relationships are built.

Picture your relationship with your wife as a garden, flourishing under the nurturing power of mutual respect. See each action, word, and choice as a seed planted in fertile soil. This soil is rich with understanding, patience, and empathy. It requires careful tending to bloom fully.

Visualize yourself and your wife standing together in this garden. You offer respect by valuing her autonomy, desires, and dreams; she provides the same in return. Together, you create a space where both of you feel seen, heard, and cherished, where your love grows without the fear of judgment or neglect.

Recognize how respect fosters an environment of trust. When respect is present, vulnerability can thrive, and each partner is free to express their needs and desires without fear of rejection or shame. You respect her in her entirety—her joy, her desires, and her choices. In turn, you honor your feelings, worth, and desires, knowing they are valid and deserve consideration.

Breathe in this deep sense of mutual respect, feeling it envelops you and your relationship. With each breath, feel more grounded in the knowing that respect is not just a foundation—it is the fuel that propels love forward, creating a stronger, more fulfilling connection with each passing day.

Affirmation:
"I honor and respect my partner in all aspects of our relationship, knowing that mutual respect deepens our connection and strengthens our love."

Practices in Action:

Activity 1: A Respectful Conversation

Set aside time to have a heart-to-heart conversation with your wife about your relationship. Discuss your needs, boundaries, and desires, and listen deeply to hers. The goal is to speak honestly while deeply respecting each other's feelings. Afterward, reflect on how this openness deepens your mutual respect.

Tip: When listening, practice empathy and refrain from interrupting. Allow space for your wife's voice as you hope she will for yours.

Activity 2: A Respect Letter

Please write a letter to your wife expressing how you respect and admire her. Focus on the qualities she possesses that you hold in high esteem—her strength, her kindness, her ability to communicate. Include specific moments when her actions or words have deepened your respect for her. Please share this letter with her when you feel the time is right.

Journaling Prompt:

Reflect on the role mutual respect plays in your relationship. How has respecting each other's autonomy and desires impacted your connection? Write about a time when you felt particularly respected by your wife, and explore how that made you feel emotionally.

Consider your actions in the relationship—how do you express respect to her in ways that honor her needs and boundaries? What are some ways you can deepen the respect you share?

Closing Reflection:

Respect is the silent strength that holds relationships together. When nurtured, it creates an atmosphere where love can grow freely, with each partner confident in the other's care and regard. Take a moment to recognize the power of mutual respect in your relationship and its profound impact on your love. As you move forward together, continue cultivating this respect, for it is the key that unlocks deeper intimacy and joy.

Embracing my feelings of love and admiration for my wife

Meditation:

Find a quiet space and settle into a comfortable position. Close your eyes and take a slow, deep breath. As you breathe in, let the air fill your lungs; as you exhale, release any tension you may be carrying. With each breath, feel yourself sinking deeper into relaxation.

Now, focus your attention on your wife. Picture her in your mind's eye—her smile, presence, and how she carries herself with grace. As you think of her, allow feelings of love and admiration to flow naturally, like a gentle wave washing over you.

Reflect on the qualities that make her so unique. Perhaps it's her strength, kindness, or ability to inspire you. Notice how, with every passing day, your admiration for her deepens, not only as your partner but as the incredible woman she is.

Visualize her thriving in her desires, her joy radiating as she grows into her full potential. You see how her happiness is intertwined with your own and how, as her partner, you contribute to the environment where she can flourish. The love you feel for her is not a possession but a celebration of who she is—a unique, assertive individual with her passions and dreams.

Breathe in this love and admiration, knowing it is not just about what she gives you but the respect and awe you hold for her. Feel gratitude for the bond you share and the opportunity to witness her joy, knowing that your love is about receiving and giving space for her to be her true self.

Affirmation:
"I embrace my love for my wife and honor her in all that she is. I admire her strength, her beauty, and the love we share."

Practices in Action:

Activity 1: Daily Expression of Admiration

Each day, take a moment to express a specific admiration for your wife. Whether it's complimenting her on her appearance, strength, or how she handles life's challenges, acknowledge the things you deeply admire about her. Please make this a part of your daily routine and share it with her genuinely and openly.

Tip: When expressing admiration, focus on her inner qualities and outer beauty. This deepens the emotional connection you share.

Activity 2: A Gratitude Journal

Take a few minutes to write in a journal, listing the qualities you admire most in your wife. Reflect on the moments when she has surprised you with her strength, wisdom, or kindness. Recognize the little things she does that might go unnoticed but mean the world to you. Afterward, share your journal entry with her if you feel comfortable, allowing her to feel the depth of your love and admiration.

Journaling Prompt:

Reflect on your feelings of love and admiration for your wife. What qualities about her do you hold in the highest regard, and how do they inspire your passion? Write about a moment when you felt particularly proud of her or in awe of her strength. How does this admiration impact your relationship, and how can you continue to celebrate her as the remarkable woman she is?

Consider how your love for her has evolved. What has deepened your appreciation for her, and how does this influence your dynamic? Explore how you can continue to support her journey and nurture the admiration that binds you.

Closing Reflection:

Love and admiration are the pillars that hold the relationship up. They create an atmosphere where both partners can thrive—one where respect and awe intertwine, creating a space for deep emotional intimacy. As you reflect on your feelings of love for your wife, take a moment to appreciate the incredible woman she is and how your admiration for her helps to foster a deeper, more fulfilling bond. Love her for what she does and who she is—entirely and unconditionally.

The thrill of sharing experiences as a couple

Meditation:

Find a quiet space, sit comfortably, and take a few deep breaths. As you inhale, let the air fill your lungs, and as you exhale, feel the weight of any tension or distractions melt away. Allow yourself to arrive fully in the present moment.

Now, think about the experiences you and your wife have shared. Picture the moments when you've connected, laughed, and found joy in each other's company. Feel the excitement of creating these shared memories, from the smallest moments to the more significant milestones in your relationship.

Visualize the two of you, side by side, growing stronger through each experience. Imagine the thrill of the adventures you've embarked on together, whether it's the joy of discoveries or the shared intimacy of deep conversations and vulnerability.

As you focus on your bond, realize that these experiences are not just shared physically but emotionally. Each encounter deepens your connection, whether exploring desires, communicating openly, or simply existing together in a moment of shared joy. Every experience is a building block that strengthens your partnership and creates a space of mutual respect and trust.

I am grateful for the opportunity to share in her happiness, knowing that these experiences aren't just about physical pleasure—they are a journey of emotional intimacy, trust, and love. The thrill lies in the moment and the depth it brings to your connection.

Affirmation:
"I celebrate the thrill of shared experiences with my wife. Our connection grows stronger with each moment we embrace together."

Practices in Action:

Activity 1: Create a New Experience Together

Choose an activity to share with your wife that neither of you has experienced before—something new that you can enjoy together, whether it's a fun outing, a new hobby, or even a new conversation about desires and boundaries. Let this new experience serve as a reminder of the excitement and connection that comes from exploring life as a couple.

Tip: Afterward, talk about how the experience made you both feel. Share your thoughts and appreciate how this new experience brought you closer.

Activity 2: Reliving a Past Experience

Look back on a moment or experience in your relationship that was particularly thrilling for both of you. Write about it in detail, focusing on the moment's emotions, connection, and excitement. Afterward, share your reflections with your wife and discuss what made that experience memorable. Discuss how these experiences shape the growth of your bond.

Journaling Prompt:

Reflect on the shared experiences that have defined your relationship. What moments stand out as particularly thrilling or deeply connecting? How do these experiences contribute to the depth of your emotional intimacy and trust? Write about a specific time when you felt excitement and connection with your wife. How did that moment affect the way you view your dynamic?

Consider how you can continue seeking out new experiences, big or small. How can you make space for ongoing adventures that deepen your bond and bring even more joy into your relationship?

Closing Reflection:

Every shared experience is a piece of the giant puzzle of your relationship, contributing to your intricate and beautiful connection with your wife. As you reflect on the thrill of these moments, let the joy, excitement, and emotional closeness you experience together remind you of the strength and depth of your partnership. Each experience you share adds to the foundation of love, respect, and intimacy that supports your relationship.

Finding peace in my role and our connection

Meditation:

Find a comfortable position and close your eyes. Take a few deep breaths, inhaling deeply through your nose and exhaling slowly through your mouth. As you breathe in, imagine filling your body with calm, and as you breathe out, release any tension or stress you may be holding onto.

Now, focus on your connection with your wife and your role within your relationship. Picture yourself standing side by side, both of you in your unique positions—partners who respect and support each other. Your role is not one of submission but one of deep trust, understanding, and love. You embrace it with pride, knowing it brings peace, strength, and growth to your connection.

Feel the peace of knowing you are where you need to be. Your role is not defined by others' opinions but by the unique bond you share with your wife. In this space, there is no judgment, only acceptance and peace.

Visualize the love and respect that flows freely between you and your wife, each embracing your role in this journey together. You are in harmony, understanding that your connection thrives because of mutual respect and shared values. The peace you feel stems from knowing that your role is valued and essential to the love and growth you both experience.

With each breath, feel more grounded in your place within your relationship. You are part of something bigger than yourself, and this knowledge brings you peace. Trust in your bond, knowing that every step you take together strengthens your emotional and spiritual connection.

Affirmation:
"I find peace in my role and my connection with my wife. Our bond is grounded in love, respect, and trust."

Practices in Action:

Activity 1: Reflect on Your Role

Take a moment to reflect on the role you play in your relationship. Write about how this role contributes to your emotional, physical, and spiritual connection with your wife. Consider how you embrace this role with pride and peace and how it enhances your love.

Tip: Remember that your role is not about comparison but what works for your unique relationship. Embrace it for what it brings to your bond.

Activity 2: Affirm Your Peace

Each morning or evening, take a moment to affirm the peace you feel in your role and your relationship. Say, "I am at peace with who I am in this relationship. My role is one of love, trust, and support." Allow yourself to feel the truth in this affirmation as you ground yourself in the peace it brings.

Journaling Prompt:

Reflect on how you feel about your role in your relationship. What aspects of your connection bring you the most peace? How does embracing your role as a cuckold contribute to the overall strength and harmony of your relationship? Write about the moments when you've felt profoundly peaceful and secure in your role and in the love you share with your wife.

How do you maintain that peace in your daily life? How can you nurture this sense of peace and balance within yourself and with your wife?

Closing Reflection:

Please take a deep breath and feel grounded in your role and the peace it brings. Your connection with your wife is unique and filled with trust, love, and respect. As you pridefully embrace your role, let the peace you feel deepen your bond and create a lasting sense of harmony. In this space of mutual understanding, you and your wife continue to grow and thrive together.

Embodying self-acceptance and growth

Meditation:

Find a quiet space and settle into a comfortable position. Close your eyes and take a few deep breaths, inhaling slowly through your nose and exhaling gently through your mouth. With each breath, feel the world's weight lift off your shoulders, allowing yourself to relax and be fully present in this moment.

Now, bring your attention to your heart. Imagine a warm light filling this space, representing your love and acceptance of yourself. See this light grow and expand as you breathe, spreading through your chest, body, and mind. This light reflects your self-acceptance, a reminder that you are worthy of love, respect, and growth.

Visualize yourself in your role, embracing it fully and with pride. Feel a deep sense of peace as you accept yourself in this relationship. Know that your role is not a limitation but a beautiful expression of trust and love between you and your partner. You do not need to be anything other than yourself, as you are loved and valued exactly as you are.

Feel the power of growth entering your body and mind with each breath. As you open yourself to new experiences and emotions, you embrace the personal development journey. You are constantly evolving, learning, and becoming more deeply connected to yourself and your partner. The growth you experience is an essential part of your relationship—individually and together.

Let go of any doubts or insecurities, knowing that self-acceptance is the key to unlocking the whole version of yourself. Embrace the growth that comes with each new experience, and trust that this journey of growth and self-love leads you toward more profound connection and understanding.

Affirmation:
"I embrace myself fully and accept my role in this relationship. I am worthy of love, growth, and acceptance, and I honor the journey of becoming the best version of myself."

Practices in Action:

Activity 1: Practice Self-Reflection

Set aside time to reflect on your journey of self-acceptance. Write about the moments when you have felt the most at peace with yourself, especially within the context of your relationship. Reflect on the growth you have experienced and how it has shaped the person you are today. This is an opportunity to acknowledge and celebrate how far you have come.

Tip: Remember, growth isn't always about grand changes—it's often found in the small, everyday actions that align with your values and bring you closer to self-acceptance.

Activity 2: Acknowledge Your Growth

Each day, take a moment to recognize one small way you've grown, either emotionally, mentally, or spiritually. Write it down and say aloud, "I am proud of the growth I've made today." Allow yourself to feel gratitude for your progress, no matter how small it may seem.

Journaling Prompt:

Reflect on how you have embraced your role and the growth that has come from it. In what ways has this journey of self-acceptance deepened your connection with your wife? Write about how you've grown, individually and as a partner, and how this growth contributes to your relationship's overall strength and harmony.

How can you continue to embrace self-acceptance moving forward? In what areas of your life do you feel you're ready to grow more deeply, and how can you invite that growth into your relationship?

Closing Reflection:

Take a deep, grounding breath, and let the sense of self-acceptance fill you. You are on a beautiful journey of growth as an individual and part of your relationship. With each step you take, you become more connected to yourself and your partner. Embrace this journey with love and trust, knowing that growth is an ongoing process that brings you closer to the most authentic version of yourself.

Seeing my wife thrive and feeling joy in that

Meditation:

Begin by finding a comfortable, relaxed position. Close your eyes and take a few deep, calming breaths. Inhale deeply through your nose, allowing your chest to expand, and exhale slowly, releasing any tension or stress from your body. With each breath, feel yourself becoming more centered and at peace.

Now, focus on your wife. Imagine her in her element—radiating confidence, happiness, and strength. Visualize her thriving in ways that bring her joy, whether in her personal life, her passions, or your relationship. See her smile, feel her energy, and know that she is flourishing in every aspect.

As you observe her thriving, allow yourself to experience the joy of seeing her happy and fulfilled fully. This joy is rooted in love and mutual respect—her growth is not separate from yours but a beautiful reflection of your connection. Know that her happiness brings you happiness; her success is yours. As she flourishes, so does the bond between you.

Feel gratitude for witnessing her growth and embrace the fulfillment from knowing she can explore her desires, passions, and full potential. There is no jealousy, only love. Her success is your success, and her joy is yours to share.

Please take a moment to bask in the warmth of this connection, the unspoken understanding that her thriving is a shared experience. You are honored to participate in her journey, offering support, trust, and unconditional love. In doing so, you also grow together.

Affirmation:
"I celebrate my wife's growth and joy and feel deep joy in her thriving. Her happiness is mine, and I am grateful for our love and support."

Practices in Action:

Activity 1: Celebrate Her Achievements

Take a moment to acknowledge and celebrate your wife's achievements, big or small. Write down three things you admire about her and how you've seen her grow or flourish recently. Reflect on how her success impacts you and the relationship, and express gratitude for your shared journey.

Tip: Express your appreciation verbally or in writing to her. Sometimes, the most straightforward words of acknowledgment can strengthen the bond between partners.

Activity 2: Support Her Growth

Think about one way to actively support your wife in her growth journey. Is there something she's been working toward that you can help with or a way you can offer emotional or practical support? Take concrete steps to show your dedication to her thriving.

Journaling Prompt:

Reflect on the joy you feel when you see your wife thriving. How does her success bring fulfillment to you? What does it feel like to see her grow, not just in the context of your relationship but in her pursuits as well? Write about how her happiness and thriving contribute to your sense of purpose and joy.

How can you continue to foster an environment where both of you are encouraged to thrive and grow together? What steps can you take to show her that her growth is something you truly celebrate?

Closing Reflection:

Take a deep breath, grounding yourself in the powerful sense of love, trust, and joy that comes from seeing your wife thrive. Embrace the beauty of her growth, knowing that her success reflects your connection. You are partners in this journey; as she flourishes, so does your bond. Continue to support, love, and celebrate her—because in doing so, you also nourish your happiness and fulfillment.

The beauty of shared pleasure and love

Meditation:

Find a comfortable, quiet space to relax in. Close your eyes and take a few deep breaths, allowing your body to settle into calm. Fill your lungs with positive energy; release tension or distractions with each exhale.

Now, focus on your connection with your wife. Imagine the moments of intimacy you've shared and the pleasure you've both experienced—physical, emotional, and mental. See how these moments have deepened your love, creating a powerful bond of trust, respect, and shared pleasure.

As you think about these shared moments, allow yourself to feel the warmth of love and gratitude. Picture yourself both together, experiencing joy, not only for your pleasure but also for your wife's pleasure. The beauty of shared pleasure is not limited to one person; it's a dynamic that brings you closer and strengthens your connection.

Feel how your satisfaction is rooted in her joy. Her pleasure is your pleasure. You are a part of each other's journey, and your happiness is intertwined. As she experiences joy, it fills your heart with fulfillment. There is no divide, only a beautiful, shared experience of love and pleasure.

Let this sense of connection grow, knowing that each shared moment of love and intimacy is a building block for a deeper, more fulfilling relationship. Your support strengthens your bond, your cherishing of her happiness, and your honoring the joy she brings into your life.

Affirmation:
"I honor the shared pleasure and love between my wife and me. Her joy and pleasure enrich my life, and we create a bond of mutual satisfaction, love, and respect together."

Practices in Action:

Activity 1: Celebrate Your Shared Intimacy

Reflect on a recent moment of shared pleasure between you and your wife. Write about the emotions you felt during that experience. How did it make you feel to see her enjoying herself? How did it deepen your connection? Reflect on the ways shared moments of pleasure enhance both of your lives.

Tip: Share these reflections with your wife, not just as a reminder of the joy you've shared, but to further build the connection and appreciation for the beauty of your mutual pleasure.

Activity 2: Create New Moments of Shared Joy

Think about something new you can do to create an experience of shared pleasure, whether physical or emotional. Maybe it's planning a particular date, a quiet moment, or an intimate gesture that will make her feel cherished. Take action and show her how much you value her pleasure and the connection you share.

Journaling Prompt:

Reflect on the role that shared pleasure plays in your relationship. How does experiencing joy together enhance your connection? Write about the sense of fulfillment you feel when both of you are satisfied and how this deepens your relationship.

How can you continue fostering this shared joy, making you feel valued and loved in every experience? What does shared pleasure look like in your relationship, and how can you nurture it moving forward?

Closing Reflection:

Take a moment to breathe deeply and reflect on the beautiful connection you share with your wife. The joy you both experience together is a testament to the love and trust that bind you. Cherish these moments of shared pleasure, knowing that they are fulfilling in the present and the foundation for a deeper, stronger relationship in the future.

Trusting the process of our evolving relationship

Meditation:

Find a comfortable space to sit or lie down, feeling relaxed and at ease. Close your eyes and take a deep breath, inhaling peace and exhaling any tension. Allow your mind to be quiet, focusing only on the rhythm of your breath as it guides you into a calm, centered place.

Now, bring your awareness to the journey you and your wife are on. Recognize that relationships are ever-evolving, growing in new directions, and adapting to your needs and desires. Imagine the trust that has been built between you, allowing your relationship to unfold naturally, without force, but with patience and respect.

See the evolution of your dynamic—how you have learned, changed, and adapted over time. You have each found your way of giving, receiving, and growing together. Trust that each step of this journey is part of a more excellent plan, one that is designed to bring you closer, deepen your connection, and enrich both of your lives.

Feel the confidence in knowing that you are moving together, not apart. The challenges you face are growth opportunities, and the moments of joy are proof of the strength of your bond. Trust in the process, trusting that it will guide you to deeper understanding, more fulfillment, and greater love.

In your heart, acknowledge that this relationship is dynamic. The love you share will continue to evolve, shifting as you both grow as individuals and as partners. Trust that, even in the uncertainty of change, there is beauty in the unfolding journey.

Affirmation:
"I trust in the evolving nature of my relationship with my wife. Each step and change is a part of our growth together, and I am confident that this journey will bring us closer, stronger, and more in love."

Practices in Action:

Activity 1: Reflecting on Growth

Take a moment to write about how your relationship has evolved since the beginning. What changes have you seen in yourself, your wife, and your dynamic? How has your understanding of each other deepened over time? Reflect on moments when you've trusted the process, even in uncertainty, and how it strengthened your bond.

Tip: Share your reflections with your wife, celebrating how far you've come and how the process has enriched both of your lives.

Activity 2: Embracing Change Together

Think about an area of your relationship that is currently evolving or changing. Please openly discuss this with your wife, acknowledging the changes and how you feel about them. Embrace the uncertainty with trust in the process, knowing that change, though sometimes uncomfortable, is a natural part of growth. Celebrate how your relationship continues to unfold in beautiful ways.

Journaling Prompt:

Write about a time when you experienced uncertainty or change in your relationship. How did you and your wife navigate it together? What did you learn about each other, and how did it strengthen your connection? How does trusting the process of evolution allow you to feel secure in your relationship moving forward?

Closing Reflection:

Sit quietly, breathe deeply, and reflect on your and your wife's journey. Recognize the trust that has carried you both through changes and challenges, and allow yourself to feel gratitude for the relationship you are building together. Trust the unfolding process, knowing that each new chapter brings you closer, not just to each other, but to your most accurate, authentic selves.

Gratitude for the deepening emotional connection

Meditation:

Find a peaceful space to relax, sitting or lying down comfortably. Close your eyes and take a slow, deep breath, inhaling deeply and exhaling fully, releasing any tension. With each breath, let go of distractions, allowing yourself to be fully present.

As you focus on your breath, bring your attention to your emotional connection with your wife. Feel the warmth and love between you, and acknowledge how this bond has deepened over time. This connection is built on trust, vulnerability, and mutual understanding—qualities that have allowed you to grow closer with each passing day.

Reflect on the moments when you've shared your emotions openly with her, when your hearts have met in a place of understanding and care. Notice how this emotional intimacy has created a strong foundation of love and how this shared space brings you comfort, joy, and fulfillment.

Feel deep gratitude for the way your relationship continues to evolve. Your bond is not static; it is a living, breathing connection that deepens when you show vulnerability, communicate openly, and support each other. This bond is a source of strength, a reminder that no matter where life takes you both, your emotional connection will remain at the heart of your shared journey.

Acknowledge how much you value the emotional depth created, and feel gratitude for your wife's openness and willingness to connect with you on such a deep and intimate level. In this moment, feel the power of this connection flow between you both and allow it to fill you with warmth and love.

Affirmation:
"I am deeply grateful for my emotional connection with my wife. Our bond continues to grow and deepen with love, trust, and understanding. I cherish this connection and the strength it brings to our relationship."

Practices in Action:

Activity 1: A Gratitude Letter

Write a heartfelt letter to your wife expressing gratitude for your shared emotional connection. Reflect on moments when you felt particularly close to her and truly understood and supported her. Let her know how much you appreciate the deep emotional intimacy that has developed between you. This will not only deepen your connection but also reinforce the gratitude you feel for each other.

Tip: Make this letter personal and specific, acknowledging how she makes you feel emotionally safe and fulfilled. It will reinforce the bond between you both.

Activity 2: Shared Emotional Reflection

Take some quiet time to reflect on how your emotional connection has grown with your wife. Discuss how you've supported each other emotionally and how you can continue to nurture this bond moving forward. Please share your thoughts on how you both feel about the emotional depth of your relationship and how it enhances your overall connection.

Journaling Prompt:

Reflect on the emotional depth you feel in your relationship. How has your connection deepened, and what experiences have contributed to that growth? How does the emotional intimacy you share make you feel supported, loved, and valued? Write about how you can continue to deepen this bond, further strengthening your connection.

Closing Reflection:

Take a moment to breathe deeply, grounded in your emotional connection with your wife. Feel the warmth of gratitude and love radiating from your heart, knowing that this bond will grow stronger with every step you take together. Trust in the deepening of your relationship, and see that it is a robust foundation to support you through all of life's changes.

Honoring the joy and love that grows between us

Meditation:

Find a quiet, comfortable place where you can relax without distractions. Close your eyes and take a slow, deep breath, feeling the air fill your lungs. As you exhale, let go of any tension in your body, allowing yourself to settle into the present moment. Breathe in deeply again, and release any remaining stress with each exhale.

Now, focus on the love and joy that have blossomed between you and your wife. Reflect on how this love has grown, not just through the moments of shared pleasure but through the bond of trust, respect, and open communication you've nurtured together. Feel the warmth of her love surrounding you and gratitude for the deepened connection with each passing day.

Visualize the joy you both experience through shared moments of intimacy, laughter, or simple connection. See how this joy radiates between you, filling your hearts with love and appreciation. The love you share is expansive, ever-growing, and filled with positive energy. It also brings fulfillment to your wife and you—because when she thrives in this dynamic, so do you.

Feel how this love continues to grow, transforming your relationship in empowering, healing, and deeply fulfilling ways. Honor the joy that fills the space between you, knowing it reflects your commitment to one another's happiness. In this dynamic, love is a living, breathing force that evolves and strengthens with time.

Acknowledge how much you cherish her happiness, knowing that her joy is the very thing that fuels your own. Allow yourself to celebrate the bond you share, a bond rooted in mutual respect, love, and the joy that flows between you both. As you honor this growth, feel the energy of that love expanding, filling your heart with peace, contentment, and profound gratitude.

Affirmation:
"I honor the joy and love that grows between us. Our bond is filled with trust, respect, and understanding. I am grateful for the love we share and the joy we both experience together."

Practices in Action:

Activity 1: Celebrating Love Together

Take time to celebrate your relationship by doing something special with your wife—whether it's a quiet evening together, a shared activity you both love, or simply enjoying each other's company in a way that brings you joy. Reflect on the moments that have deepened your love and connection. Make a conscious effort to celebrate the love growing between you.

Tip: Create a small ritual of appreciation, whether sharing a moment of gratitude each day or simply taking time to be present together. This will help nurture the love and joy you've cultivated.

Activity 2: Reflecting on the Journey

Reflect on how far you've come in your relationship. Write about the ways your love has evolved and deepened over time. What moments have stood out as turning points in your emotional connection? Celebrate how much you've grown as individuals and partners, and express gratitude for the joy born from your shared journey.

Journaling Prompt:

Write about the love that has blossomed between you and your wife. How has this love grown and deepened? What moments have made you feel incredibly grateful for the joy that flows between you both? How does honoring her happiness and shared experiences enhance your fulfillment and joy? Write about how you can continue to nurture and celebrate this love as it grows.

Closing Reflection:

Take a moment to breathe deeply and reflect on the growth of love in your relationship. Feel the peace and joy that come from honoring the love you share, and know that this connection will continue to evolve and thrive. Celebrate the beauty of your bond, and feel gratitude for the joy, love, and fulfillment it brings. You are both contributing to a love that is expansive, empowering, and deeply meaningful.

Rachel, Michael, and David: A Rare Love

The Interview

Before we dive into our three participants' intimate and personal experiences, it's important to note that the following interview is entirely fictional. The individuals sharing their stories are not real people, but their experiences are meant to represent a deeper exploration of the emotions, connections, and dynamics that can exist within the unique hotwife, cuckold, and bull relationship.

This interview is not meant to be a "how-to" guide or a step-by-step manual for anyone looking to enter this dynamic. Instead, it serves as a window into the hearts and minds of those who have embraced this unconventional relationship structure, showing the love, trust, and mutual respect that underpin their choices. The goal is to offer insight into the human experience of navigating these roles and exploring the complexities, joys, and emotional growth of embracing a relationship that challenges traditional norms.

As you read through the interview, remember that these are the stories of fictional characters. They speak from a place of openness and vulnerability, sharing their journeys of discovery, growth, and connection. Their experiences may not mirror your own, but they aim to offer a sense of understanding, validation, and inspiration for anyone curious about or involved in a similar dynamic.

Now, let's listen to the voices of these three individuals—each with their own perspective and experiences—and share what it means to love, trust, and support one another in a relationship built on openness and respect.

Introduction

In the complex landscape of modern relationships, what does it mean to love, respect, and honor one another? What happens when boundaries are respected and celebrated and when emotional connection is valued as much as physical desire? Today, we meet three individuals whose lives are bound by these principles, navigating a dynamic that challenges traditional labels while embracing mutual respect, trust, and profound connection.

Rachel, Michael, and David share a unique and profoundly fulfilling relationship—a marriage where love is the foundation, but freedom, exploration, and emotional growth play vital roles. While Rachel and Michael have been married for ten years, their connection has evolved in ways that many might find unconventional, but for them, it is the most accurate form of love and trust.

Rachel is what some might call a "hotwife," a term that in their relationship is less about a physical act and more about a profound emotional understanding: Rachel is encouraged to explore her sexual freedom, always with the unwavering support of her husband, Michael. Their relationship thrives because of their open communication, mutual respect, and deep love. Michael's role is one of support and admiration, finding joy in seeing his wife thrive in both love and lust, confident that their emotional bond will always be the strongest.

David, who shares an intimate connection with Rachel, is not just a participant in their marriage; he is a cherished and respected part of their lives. His role within this relationship is one of deep emotional intimacy and trust. This person respects the boundaries set by both Rachel and Michael and values the love they all share. His connection with them isn't just about physical attraction but the emotional bond and respect they've built over time.

Together, they represent a family not defined by traditional expectations but by love, respect, and open communication. Their relationship is a testament to what can be created when partners are free to be themselves and supported by each other in their personal growth and desires.

In this interview, we will hear from each of them, gaining insight into how their relationship functions, how they navigate the complexities of their dynamic, and how each person finds fulfillment in their unique connection. From Rachel's journey of empowerment and exploration to Michael's deep love and understanding of his role as a supportive husband to David's respectful and nurturing involvement, we will uncover the layers of this modern family, built on trust, love, and mutual respect.

Rachel

Rachel, thank you so much for agreeing to sit down and talk with us today. How did this dynamic develop in your relationship with Michael?

Rachel: Thank you for having me. We did not initially set out to explore it, but it evolved naturally. Michael and I have been together for over a decade, and our relationship has always been grounded in trust and open communication. We were always comfortable discussing our feelings, needs, and desires from the start. That transparency has always been our biggest strength.

In the early years of our marriage, we were like any other couple, just trying to make things work. We loved each other profoundly and permanently and felt like we were growing together. But there came a point when we realized that our love wasn't just about sharing our everyday lives; it was about supporting each other's growth in all areas. That's when the conversation about exploring new dynamics first started. We were curious about what freedom and exploration could look like for us as a couple and how we could deepen our connection, not just emotionally but also sexually.

Michael was the one who first brought up the idea of me exploring outside of our relationship safely and lovingly. We were both surprised by how natural the conversation felt. The idea didn't threaten him—he seemed excited for me to explore and find pleasure in new ways. That trust he showed me in that moment is something I'll never forget. It was a turning point. From there, we began researching and learning about the "hotwife" dynamic, and it felt like it was something we could embrace together. We weren't just following a trend; we were creating something that felt authentic to who we are.

That's beautiful. It sounds like trust has been a massive part of your journey. How has this dynamic strengthened your relationship with Michael?

Rachel: Trust is everything, yes. I honestly think the biggest thing it's done is bring us closer. We communicate more openly now than we ever have before. Michael knows I'll always come to him with my feelings about our dynamic or something else. We've been able to talk about our needs and desires in a way that feels healthy and open. There's this fantastic freedom in knowing that I have his full support. It doesn't mean there aren't moments of vulnerability or uncertainty, but we always work through them together.

The emotional intimacy we've built through this has deepened our connection in ways I never imagined. And I also feel this beautiful sense of pride when I'm with Michael. I'm proud of our relationship and the trust that we've built. We've never been more in love, and we've never been more connected. It's as if our bond has grown stronger with every new layer we add. This dynamic isn't just about me exploring—I've always felt it's *our* journey.

That's moving. You also mentioned that David is a part of this dynamic. How does he fit into your relationship with Michael, and how has that connection shaped your experiences?

Rachel: David is an essential part of our lives. It's about the physical connection and the emotional bond we've all built. From the very first time I met David, there was this understanding between all three of us. He wasn't just someone I was seeing outside of my marriage—he was someone who respected our relationship and cared for us both deeply. His role in this is one of trust and respect, just like Michael's. It's never been about competition or insecurity; it's always been about shared experiences and love.

For me, being with David is about feeling empowered in my sexuality, but it's also about feeling the support and love of both men. It's not about filling a void in my relationship with Michael—it's about adding to it. Every experience I've shared with David has made me feel more confident and connected to them. I can see how much Michael enjoys seeing me happy and fulfilled, and I think that's one of the most beautiful parts of our dynamic. Michael's joy comes from knowing that I'm thriving and experiencing pleasure.

David, too, has always shown respect for the emotional bond that Michael and I share. It's never been about trying to take anything away from our marriage—it's about celebrating the love we all share. The three of us have become a family, and I genuinely believe that love has only grown because of how we've approached this dynamic with openness and mutual respect.

This dynamic is built on respect, love, and trust. How do you think this experience impacted your sense of self and relationship with your desires?

Rachel: Honestly, it's been a journey of self-discovery. I've always been a confident person, but being able to explore my sexuality in such an open and supportive way has helped me embrace my desires in a more profound, more authentic way. I've learned so much about myself—what I enjoy, what excites me, and what makes me feel truly alive. But more than that, I've learned that my desires are valid. I don't have to suppress or hide any part of myself. I'm allowed to experience joy, to be free, and to explore without guilt.

It's also made me realize just how important it is to have a partner who is fully supportive of your journey, who doesn't just accept your desires but encourages you to explore them. Michael has always respected my need for independence and self-expression, which is why this dynamic works well for us. It's not about one partner feeling like they're giving up something—it's about mutual respect and creating space for both people to grow.

Finally, Rachel, how would you describe your love for Michael and David? Each of you brings something unique to the relationship.

Rachel: I love both of them deeply. Michael is my rock, my partner, the love of my life. He's the one who's always there for me, who supports me no matter what. My love for him is unshakeable, and how he shows me daily how much he cares—whether through a word of encouragement or a quiet gesture—means everything to me. I can't imagine my life without him.

As for David, there's a different kind of love, one rooted in mutual respect and admiration. We share something that goes beyond the physical—it's about emotional connection and trust. I feel so grateful to have both of these amazing men in my life, and the love we share isn't just about the moments we're together—it's about how we all grow together.

Our relationship has a unique beauty that I can't quite explain. But when we are together, I feel I'm exactly where I'm meant to be. It's a deep, expansive love built on the most vital foundation of trust, respect, and mutual admiration.

<u>**David**</u>

David, thank you for being here. You're part of an unconventional relationship dynamic, and I'm sure many people are curious about what that looks like. Can you share how you came to be involved with Rachel and Michael?

David: Absolutely, and thank you for having me. When I first met Michael and Rachel, I had no idea that something like this would evolve. We started as friends, just getting to know each other, and we clicked immediately. There was an instant connection, and the chemistry was undeniable. Over time, Michael and Rachel shared their relationship dynamic with me, and I was genuinely intrigued. They both made it clear from the start that they were looking for someone who would respect their bond and the love they shared but also someone who could add to their journey. I remember Michael expressing how much he wanted Rachel to experience joy and pleasure outside of their relationship, and that's when it hit me—that this was about more than just a physical connection. It was about building something meaningful, rooted in respect and trust.

From there, things progressed naturally. Rachel and I developed a strong emotional connection, and we've all worked hard to ensure this dynamic is fulfilling for everyone involved. It's never been about "stepping in" or "taking over." It's about supporting Rachel and Michael and helping create a space where all of us can thrive.

That's an insightful way of describing it. Your role in this dynamic seems to be one of respect and support. How has that relationship with both Michael and Rachel evolved?

David: That's precisely it—respect and support. Honestly, the more time we've spent together, the more I've come to appreciate the unique bond that Michael and Rachel share. Their relationship is grounded in trust, and that's something that makes everything work so well. Being involved in their dynamic has been about more than just the physical side—it's been about emotional connections, open communication, and mutual respect.

Over time, we've all grown closer as friends and partners in this arrangement. There's much love between the three of us. I don't see myself as just an "outside" presence in their relationship—I'm a part of the woven fabric between us all. The fact that we all share in this journey with openness and understanding has made our connection stronger. I feel deeply honored to be able to contribute to their happiness and fulfillment.

You have a lot of respect for the relationship that Michael and Rachel have built. How has being part of this dynamic impacted your views on relationships and love?

David: It's been a transformative experience, honestly. I had a traditional view of relationships before I met Michael and Rachel. I always considered love as something between two people—monogamous and exclusive. But being involved in this dynamic has opened my eyes to the possibility that love doesn't have to be confined to one set structure.

I've learned that love is about connection, respect, and trust. It's about being there for the people you care about and supporting them in their journey. I've seen how Michael's love for Rachel is unwavering and how Rachel's love for Michael grows stronger with each new experience. That kind of love—where you can love someone freely, without fear or jealousy—is extraordinary. It's something that I've come to admire deeply.

This dynamic has taught me the value of emotional depth. It's not just about physical pleasure; it's about sharing moments, being vulnerable, and creating a bond beyond the surface. I've come to appreciate how much emotional intimacy plays a role. It's the foundation of everything we do together. None of this would work without that trust or emotional connection.

It sounds like a deep and meaningful experience. How would you describe your love and respect for Rachel and Michael?

David: The love I feel for Rachel and Michael is profound. It's not the typical kind of love you might read about in fairy tales, but it's genuine. With Rachel, we've built something beautiful—there's plenty of passion, but a deep emotional connection has also strengthened over time. She's an incredible woman, and being with her is a gift. I admire her confidence, her ability to be open, and her ability to love so deeply.

As for Michael, my respect for him runs deep. It takes incredible trust and security to embrace a dynamic like this. It's not something everyone could do, but Michael has never let his insecurity or jealousy get in the way of what we've all built. He's supported me in every step of this journey, and I think that's what makes this dynamic work so well. It's not about ownership; it's about sharing. And Michael has made it clear that he's fully invested in Rachel's happiness, which I deeply respect.

It is refreshing to hear about a relationship dynamic based on trust and mutual respect. Finally, David, what would you say is the most rewarding aspect of being a part of this relationship?

David: The most rewarding part is seeing the joy and fulfillment we all experience—Rachel, Michael, and myself. There's nothing more satisfying than knowing that you're contributing to someone else's happiness, especially in such a positive and healthy way. I've seen Rachel flourish in ways I didn't think were possible, and knowing that I played a role in that is incredibly fulfilling. And for Michael, watching his wife thrive and sharing in that joy is just beautiful. There's no competition here. We're all in this together, and shared happiness and love is the most rewarding thing for me.

It's also gratifying to see the strength of their bond. It reminds me that love is so much bigger than we often think. It can expand, evolve, and bring people together in the most unexpected ways. Being a part of this has indeed been a privilege.

<u>Michael</u>

Michael, thank you for being here and sharing your story. From what I understand, you and Rachel share a profound connection, but your relationship also includes another unique dynamic. Could you share how you invited another person, like David, into your relationship?

Michael: Absolutely, and thank you for taking the time to hear our story. Rachel and I have been together for a long time, and our bond is powerful—there's no doubt about that. We love each other deeply, and we've always been open and communicative about our feelings, desires, and the things that fulfill us. But over time, I could tell something was missing from Rachel. I noticed a longing in her eyes—a desire for more.

It wasn't that she wasn't happy in our relationship—she was—but I could sense that she needed something that I couldn't provide, at least not how she needed it. I wasn't sure exactly what that was at first, but I could tell she was yearning for something deeper, something different. And as much as it stung to admit it, I knew that I wasn't the one who could fully satisfy that need.

We had always been very open about our fantasies and desires, so one day, after talking it through, Rachel shared her thoughts with me. She wanted to explore being with another man, and it wasn't about me not being enough. It was about her wanting to experience something new and find a connection with someone else that she could share with me.

At first, I was hesitant. There was a lot to consider, and I wasn't sure if I was ready. But I realized that this wasn't about me not being enough but about Rachel's happiness and fulfillment. And in the end, that's what mattered to me most.

It sounds like you made this decision carefully and thoughtfully. How did you both select the right person to join you?

Michael: That's an essential part of this. Rachel and I wanted to ensure we invited someone to respect our dynamic and relationship. This wasn't about just anyone joining us—it was about finding someone who could contribute to Rachel's joy and our connection.

We met a couple of guys before David, and while they were friendly, I could tell that Rachel didn't have that spark. It wasn't anything against them; it just wasn't a match. But when we met David, it was different. There was this natural chemistry, and I could see how Rachel responded to him. He respected our boundaries and was open about his feelings, making it clear that he was fit for what we sought.

I also appreciate that David sees this dynamic as we do—it's not just about physical pleasure. It's about the emotional connection, the trust, and the understanding that we're all here to support each other. That's why our relationship works so well—we all see the value in what we're building together.

That's a mature and thoughtful approach to this. In your role, how do you balance your love and support for Rachel with your connection to David?

Michael: It's an interesting balance, for sure. The way I look at it is that my love for Rachel hasn't changed. If anything, it's deepened. Knowing she's happy and seeing her experience joy and pleasure with someone else makes me happy. But I also don't see it as me taking a step back or stepping down—I'm not any less of a partner to her, and I'm not any less of a man. It's not about dominance or submission in any traditional sense; it's about recognizing her needs and supporting them in whatever way I can.

I wouldn't describe myself as "submissive" to Rachel—I'm still very much her equal in our relationship. But in this specific context, my role is to be supportive, to encourage her to be open, and to experience what makes her feel alive and fulfilled. And that's what I've done. It's about respect. It's about honoring her desires. I don't think that diminishes my masculinity in any way; if anything, it takes strength to be secure in yourself and be open to this kind of arrangement.

And with David, there's this mutual respect. We have a relationship that's built on trust and clear boundaries. I know where I stand and that David respects Rachel and me as a couple. It's not about competition—it's about shared happiness.

You've embraced this dynamic with love and understanding. How would you describe the most rewarding aspect of it?

Michael: The most rewarding part for me is seeing Rachel truly thrive. I can see how much joy this brings her, and knowing I played a part in that fulfillment is incredibly gratifying. Rachel's confidence, excitement, and happiness shine through, and it's honestly the most fulfilling feeling. There's much freedom in seeing her live her truth and knowing that we're building something special together.

At the same time, it's rewarding to see the trust between all of us grow. There's no jealousy here, no insecurity. We're all in this together, and that bond is so strong. And honestly, it's been eye-opening for me. It's not just about "letting someone else into our bed"; it's about creating something bigger than just a relationship. It's about community, respect, and love.

It's incredible to hear how much love and respect permeate everything you've shared. Finally, Michael, what advice would you give someone considering a dynamic like yours?

Michael: My most extensive advice would be approaching it with an open heart and mind. You can't do this out of fear, jealousy, or insecurity. It has to come from a place of trust and mutual respect. Communication is vital—without it, none of this would work. And lastly, always put the happiness and well-being of your partner first. If you can, you're setting the foundation for something extraordinary.

What we've built with David is something special, and it's because we approached it with care, understanding, and lots of love. That's what makes it work. It's about trust, being open to growth, and honoring each other's journey. If you can do that, you'll have something compelling.

<u>**Closing**</u>

What a remarkable journey you've shared with us today. Thank you, Rachel, Michael, and David, for your openness and allowing us to step inside the unique dynamic you've built together. Before we close, I'd like to ask you to reflect on what you hope others can take away from your story.

Rachel: The biggest thing for me is the importance of authenticity. We all deserve to be ourselves in our relationships. It's not about fitting into someone else's expectations—it's about finding a partner who respects and supports who you are at your core. David and Michael have allowed me to explore and feel genuinely seen and loved. I hope people take away that when you trust your partner and yourself, you can create something beautiful together, no matter how unconventional it seems.

David: For me, it's about trust and mutual respect. What we've built isn't about dominance or control—it's about honoring each other's needs and desires. Conventional norms don't restrict the love we share; it's deeper and more fulfilling because we're all allowed to be our true selves. I think that's the key—communicating openly and without judgment and being willing to grow together. That's the foundation of a loving relationship, and it's been a gift to experience it with Rachel and Michael.

Michael: I agree with both of them. I've learned through this experience that love can take on many different shapes, and that's okay. I never thought I'd be in a relationship like this, but it's made me grow in ways I never expected. I've learned that love is not about possession—it's about connection, trust, and giving the people you care about the freedom to explore and experience life to its fullest. I hope people see that a fulfilling relationship doesn't look the same for everyone, but that doesn't make it any less meaningful.

That was beautifully said. Your bond is clearly rooted in trust, respect, and a deep love for one another, and that's something we can all learn from. Thank you again for sharing your story with us. We wish you continued growth and happiness as you write your story together.